Yoga

Discipline of Freedom

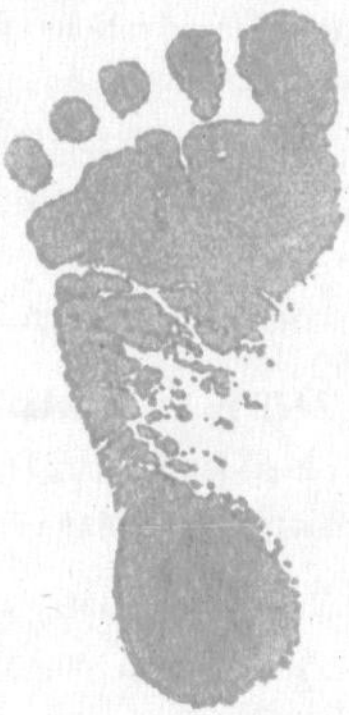

Bantam Wisdom Editions

New Translations and Interpretations of Ancient and Sacred Texts

TAO TE CHING:
The Classic Book of Integrity and the Way
Lao Tzu
TRANSLATED BY VICTOR H. MAIR

THE BHAGAVAD-GITA:
Krishna's Counsel in Time of War
TRANSLATED BY BARBARA STOLER MILLER

I CHING:
A New Interpretation for Modern Times
SAM REIFLER

THE BOOK OF FIVE RINGS
MIYAMOTO MUSASHI

THE TIBETAN BOOK OF THE DEAD
TRANSLATED BY ROBERT A. F. THURMAN

VISIONS OF GOD:
Four Medieval Mystics and Their Writings
KAREN ARMSTRONG

DHAMMAPADA:
The Sayings of Buddha
THOMAS CLEARY

Yoga

Discipline of Freedom

The *Yoga Sutra* Attributed to Patanjali

A translation of the text, with commentary,
introduction, and glossary of keywords

by Barbara Stoler Miller

BANTAM BOOKS

New York Toronto London Sydney Auckland

YOGA: DISCIPLINE OF FREEDOM
A Bantam Book/March 1998

PUBLISHING HISTORY

University of California Press hardcover edition / 1996
Bantam trade paperback edition / March 1998

Cover art by Marcia Lippman

Library of Congress Cataloging Card Number: 96-23393

ISBN 0-553-37428-1

Published simultaneously in the United States and Canada

Bantam Books are published by Bantam Books, a division of Random House, Inc.
Its trademark, consisting of the words "Bantam Books" and the portrayal of a rooster, is Registered in U.S. Patent and Trademark Office and in other countries. Marca Registrada.
Bantam Books, 1540 Broadway, New York, New York 10036.

Printed in the United States of America
10 9 8 7 6

Again, for Gwenn,
at the point of calm

CONTENTS

PREFACE

At the heart of all meditative practice in Asia is what Indians call *yoga,* the system that "yokes" one's consciousness to a spiritually liberating discipline. In his *Yoga Sutra* the ancient Indian philosopher Patanjali presents us with the possibility of complete psychological transformation through the discipline of yoga. Each of the 195 aphorisms that constitute the *Yoga Sutra* is part of Patanjali's scheme for radically altering our conception of the world and the structure of thought through which we relate to it. The text is neither a sacred scripture nor a historical artifact, but a set of philosophical analyses that probe timeless dilemmas of cognition and obstacles to spiritual tranquility. Patanjali is not engaged in a search for new knowledge. Rather, he seeks a new perspective on the nature of knowing—a way to clear the mind of accumulated experiences and memories that bind us to a world of pain.

Yogic practice culminates in a state of spiritual freedom, an absolute calm beyond the realm of language and everyday experience. Although the freedom of yoga cannot be grasped by ordinary knowledge, it is not realized through mystical experience but through a logical series of meditative practices and hyperconscious thought experiments. Patanjali's method for achieving insight is far from the mystical ecstasy of a poet like St. John of the Cross or the ritual ecstasy of a shaman in a trance. It is instead a contemplative intensity that unbinds the constraints of everyday experience.

Yoga was known to the West in ancient times, but it gained wide attention in Europe and America only in the nineteenth century, first through the *Bhagavad Gita* and later through Patanjali's *Yoga Sutra*. In Europe, Wilhelm Friedrich Hegel, who was introduced to yoga through the philological studies of Wilhelm von Humbolt, considered it to be the central teaching of the *Bhagavad Gita* and therefore to represent the core of Indian religion and philosophy. In America, Ralph Waldo Emerson and Henry David Thoreau were also deeply interested in the yoga of the *Bhagavad Gita*. In an 1849 letter to a friend, Thoreau wrote that he was, in his way, striving to practice "the yoga" faithfully and concluded that at "rare intervals, even I am a yogi." While Thoreau's practical interest in yoga was consonant with his own ascetic and contemplative experiments, the rigors of yogic practice remained daunting to less-committed Westerners.

Yoga entered the public imagination in America a century ago in the person of an Indian yogi, Swami Vivekananda. The highly educated scion of a distinguished Bengali family, in his youth Vivekananda became a disciple of the Hindu mystic Ramakrishna, acknowledged throughout India as a saintly yogi. Before he died in 1886, Ramakrishna instructed his young disciple to carry his teachings into the world. In 1893 Vivekananda electrified the World Parliament of Religions at its meeting in Chicago with his speech on what he called *raja-yoga,* the "royal yoga." It was based on Patanjali's *Yoga Sutra,* as interpreted by Ramakrishna. In 1894 Vivekananda initiated classes in New York on the Yoga school and on Vedanta, the dominant Hindu monistic philosophy rooted in ancient Vedic teachings. During a second visit to the United States in 1899, he founded the New York Vedanta Society and gave talks on *raja-yoga,* which were published by the Society in a series of Vivekananda's teachings. The volume on *raja-yoga* is a translation of Patanjali's work, with Vivekananda's commentary. Within the extensive body of Vivekananda's teachings on Yoga and Vedanta, his commentary on the devotional and service aspects of yoga supplement Patanjali's philosophical and meditative emphases. Many modern translations and commentaries on the *Yoga Sutra* reflect Vivekananda's Vedantic conceptions, among them the well-known version of Christopher Isherwood and Swami Prabhavananda, entitled "How to Know God." Isherwood, a British writer, was a great admirer of Vivekananda and a supporter of the Vedanta Society in California. Prabhavananda was a monk in the Vedanta lineage of Vivekananda.

The practice of postures, known as *haṭha-yoga,* was given minimal attention by Vivekananda as the least important component of yogic practice. Even so, this physical dimension has been extremely popular in the West and is widely practiced as a way to promote health and mental tranquility. Although few practitioners venture into the philosophical landscape of Patanjali, his analysis of human thought processes underlies the teachings of most of the gurus of yoga who have come from India.

My own interest in Patanjali's text dates back more than twenty-five years, to when I read it as one of the foundation texts of Indian philosophy. As a philosophy student I was intrigued by the startling ways in which Patanjali analyzed epistemological problems and by the method of practice he offered to penetrate them. I have tried to practice yoga ever since. More recently, my work on the *Bhagavad Gita* focused my attention on the concept of yoga and drew me back to Patanjali. An attempt to teach the *Yoga Sutra* through extant translations convinced me of the need to rescue the text from the overly technical language and scholastic debates that obscure Patanjali's brilliant analysis of how the workings of thought trap us in misconceptions about ourselves and the world. I also saw the need to find consistent equivalents in English for Patanjali's core vocabulary, rather than perpetuating the loose array of incomprehensible technical inventions on which translators have too often relied. Furthermore, disputed meanings in the commentaries are frequently muddied in translation. For example, the keyword *citta,* which most translators and commentators render as "mind," is a major source of confusion. According to Patanjali mind is but one component of the mental structure, so I translate *citta* as "thought" and maintain this distinction, as well as many others, in keeping with Patanjali's precision. I have appended a glossary that shows every occurrence of each keyword in Patanjali's system, thus enabling the reader to grasp the meaning of the term in its various contexts. As a further aid to comprehending the *Yoga Sutra,* I have grouped the aphorisms into logical sections and commented on each group.

My commentary draws on traditional Indian commentaries. But rather than argue with the scholastics, I have made it my primary purpose to clarify the meaning of each aphorism from within the text. The meaning behind and within the technical references and arguments of certain sutras is highly controversial and is debated in the traditional commentaries. To penetrate most of these debates demands a control of the Sanskrit language and of the sources of Patanjali's ideas in Vedic, Buddhist, Jain, and epic literature. Fortunately, the basic insights offered in the *Yoga Sutra* have a self-referential clarity that is independent of knowledge outside the text.

The text is in places highly technical, but not uniformly so. Not all sutras are equal in importance or in the complexity of their technical references and implied arguments. My translation is an attempt to make Patanjali's profound insights into the possibility of human spiritual freedom accessible to anyone intent on pondering the ideas of this ancient teaching.

I am grateful to the late Royal Weiler, in whose Sanskrit class I first read the *Yoga Sutra,* where it was considered not only in terms of the traditional commentaries but also in the context of Buddhist psychology. It was my editor and friend Toni Burbank who urged me to make this basic text of Indian philosophy accessible to educated American readers. For their insights and critical comments on various versions of my translation and commentary, I thank Collett Cox, Madeleine Gins, Orrin Hein, Eric Huberman, Matthew Kapstein, Fred Smith, and my husband, Maxwell Greenwood. My final reading of the text has been deepened by the questions of students who struggled with me to unravel the meaning of Patanjali's dense Sanskrit aphorisms.

Barbara Stoler Miller
New York, August 1992

INTRODUCTION

The aim of yoga is to eliminate the control that material nature exerts over the human spirit, to rediscover through introspective practice what the poet T. S. Eliot called the "still point of the turning world." This is a state of perfect equilibrium and absolute spiritual calm, an interior refuge in the chaos of worldly existence. In the view of Patanjali, yogic practice can break habitual ways of thinking and acting that bind one to the corruptions of everyday life. Although the practice of yoga is much more ancient than the *Yoga Sutra,* this brief text represents the earliest known systematic statement of the philosophical insights and practical psychology that define yoga. Through the centuries since its composition, it has been reinterpreted to meet the needs of widely divergent schools of Indian yoga, for which it remains an essential text.

More broadly, yoga refers to the complex system of physical and spiritual disciplines that is fundamental to Buddhist, Jain, and Hindu religious practice throughout Asia. The meditating figures of the Buddha and the Hindu god Shiva are familiar images in Asian religion. Sculptures show the Buddha seated in calm repose teaching his doctrine of universal compassion and the ascetic god Shiva in postures of perfect discipline. Hindu poets also evoke Shiva in his Himalayan retreat seated cross-legged and completely motionless, absorbed in pure contemplation, like an ocean without waves, the gates of his mind closed to outside intrusion as he meditates on the self within himself.[1]

These descriptions suggest the physical and psychological state of an adept who follows the path prescribed in the *Yoga Sutra.* For Patanjali, physical control is only a precondition of inner spiritual perfection, which is cultivated by confronting the paradoxical nature of memory and thought itself. His analysis exposes the mechanisms whereby we construct false identities and enslave ourselves to a world of pain.

In our time, with its bewildering complexity and seductive material culture, Patanjali's system of yoga offers a set of powerful techniques for countering the tyranny of private mental chaos and moral confusion. Personal freedom is the concern normally associated with the private sphere, and morality with the public sphere. But they are inseparable. In the ancient Indian hierarchy of values, a concern with ultimate spiritual freedom is dominant, and yet the discipline that is required to achieve freedom is rooted in moral behavior, according to Patanjali.[2] Even though proper moral action in the world is not the goal of yoga, a great vow to live by the universal principles of nonviolence, truthfulness, avoidance of stealing, celibacy, and poverty is specified as a precondition for further yogic practice (2.30–31). The cultivation of friendship, compassion, joy, and impartiality toward all creatures, a central formula of Buddhist ethics, is also deemed efficacious for achieving the absolute tranquility of yoga (1.33). The antiworldly isolation prescribed for certain stages of yoga is not the ultimate yogic state. Periods of solitude are necessary, but one need not renounce the world forever in order to practice yoga. Indian, Chinese, and Japanese thinkers have for centuries emphasized that the spiritually liberated person can be a powerful moral force in the world. Such contemporary figures as the present Dalai Lama of Tibet and the Burmese leader Aung San Suu Kyi exemplify this possibility.

In the Indian view, the practitioner of yoga is not a passive person, but a spiritual hero who is active and potent. A sense of what it means to be a real adept in yoga can be gleaned from the parable of the princess Chudala, an extraordinary beauty who was married in her youth to a neighboring prince and who later became his spiritual teacher. In Indian culture, it is not unusual to hear of loving couples who turn to spiritual pursuits when the pleasures of the flesh wane, nor is it rare for a woman to achieve spiritual perfection. And so it was with Chudala and her husband.[3] Chudala spent all her time in study and meditation, gaining a deep calm and insight that left her husband bewildered. Against his sage wife's advice that spiritual peace was not to be found in external circumstances, he decided to renounce his kingdom and retreat to the distant forest. In his absence she ruled the country.

Through her yogic practice, Chudala had acquired great psychic and physical powers. She could take any form she chose and project it by means of her thought. She assumed the form of a young ascetic, who appeared before her husband as he wandered in the forest, and offered herself as his teacher. She instructed him in meditation and mind control, and then withdrew to let him practice. He achieved a state of pure contemplation (*samādhi*) and annihilated the wild bird of his mind—but as a result he withdrew even further from the world.

Nonetheless, Chudala persisted, using her yogic powers to enter her husband's body and awaken him from within, coaxing him back into the mundane world. In order to instruct him further, she then assumed various guises to test the true depth of his spiritual accomplishment. Convinced that his equanimity was firm, she led him back to fulfill his kingly duties with a spiritual detachment that would benefit the world. Indeed, in the strictest sense yoga is the absolute detachment of one's spirit from the corruptions of the material world, an interior freedom from the insidious cycles of desire, anger, and delusion.

The parable is consonant with Patanjali's exposure of the multiple paradoxes in the human quest for spiritual freedom. On a simple level, the desire for freedom provides the motivation to undertake the arduous discipline of yoga, but this desire itself is a potential obstacle to freedom: it must be transcended. The quest for absolute perfection is hampered by the time-bound conventions according to which we conceptualize the human condition.[4] To grasp the paradox of the spirit's limitation we have to pare away layers of misunderstanding, using thought to experience and overcome the limitations of thought itself. Recognizing the paradoxical nature of things is fundamental to breaking the connections between fragments of experience and obliterating the constructs of memory, which give an illusion of permanent identity to "individuals" and "events."

From Patanjali's perspective, the ultimate truth of the human condition cannot be known rationally, because this truth is elusive, and any attempt to objectify it can delude us. Within the practice of yoga, rational knowledge is necessary in order to proceed, but this knowledge is only conditional and experimental. Even meditation and certain levels of pure contemplation are based on past experiences that leave traces, which Patanjali calls "seeds" (*bīja;* 1.41–46). Contemplation without seeds (*nirbīja-samādhi*) is a hyperconscious condition in which thought is tranquil and totally integrated, so that it leaves no seeds to mature into further thoughts. In seed-bearing contemplation, the knowledge that spirit and material nature are fundamentally distinct is acquired through rational and intuitive means, which depend on memory. When this knowledge is realized directly, without intellectual activity, however, the result is seedless contemplation. Past experiences recorded in memory have no relevance in seedless contemplation, where all thought ceases and the spirit is completely free from the material world (1.47–51).

Patanjali's conception of freedom is related to the ancient Buddhist view that the source of suffering is the craving for permanence in a universe of impermanence, which encourages a false belief in an enduring individual self.[5] Attachment to life is so powerful that it afflicts even those who intellectually understand the transience of all things—unless they are disciplined in yoga. However, Patanjali's worldview differs significantly from that of the Buddhists in his belief in an idealized state of undifferentiated cosmic equilibrium between two enduring primal principles, spirit (*puruṣa*) and material nature (*prakṛti*). In this state, spirit is absolutely distinct from material nature and is free within itself. Buddhists, by contrast, insist on the absence of any enduring entity, spiritual or material.

The enigma of spiritual freedom is contained within the word *yoga* itself. *Yoga* is a Sanskrit word, cognate with the English word *yoke* with which it shares its most basic meanings. Yoga means "yoking" in the sense of spiritual discipline that requires preparatory exercises to gain control of the body, senses, and mind. It may also mean "integration," referring to the spiritual integrity of the individual and the cosmos. In the *Yoga Sutra,* yoga refers both to a process of discipline and its goal. It is the entire process that enables one to realize a state of absolute spiritual integration, which is freedom. Freedom is thus the result of experience rather than mere knowledge; it is an enlightening realization, not a separate phenomenon that knowledge produces.

The essential assumption underlying yogic practice is that the true state of the human spirit is freedom, which has been lost through misidentification of one's place in a phenomenal world of ceaseless change. This is the root of human suffering. Paradoxically, in yoga the freedom of spiritual integrity occurs in the act of discipline itself, which is ultimately rendered superfluous by the reality its practice discloses.

THE COMPOSITION AND CONTEXT OF THE *YOGA SUTRA*

Historical evidence regarding the authorship and the time of the composition of the *Yoga Sutra* is lacking. The dating of the text varies by centuries, but the majority of scholars consider it to have been composed around the third century A.D., a conclusion based on textual analysis of ideas common to the *Yoga Sutra* and other Hindu, Jain, and Buddhist works, including the *Bhagavad Gita.* Most would also agree not only on its status as the earliest extant codification of yogic analysis and practice but also that the original text considerably antedates the philosophical commentary on it composed by Vyasa in the eighth century A.D.

Some students of the *Yoga Sutra* would date it as early as the third century B.C. on the basis of attempts to identify its author with the Patanjali who wrote an important Sanskrit grammatical text, the *Mahabhashya,* which dates to the second century B.C.[6] There are also scattered references to other works attributed to an author named Patanjali. The attributions are linked by a legend that makes Patanjali (like Caraka, the author of the oldest system of classical Hindu medicine) an incarnation of the mythical serpent Ananta or Shesha, on whom the god Vishnu rests before the beginning of a new cycle of creation. This serpent took on human form in order to write under the name of Patanjali for the benefit of mankind.[7]

The legend is further elaborated to explain the name Patanjali. The author is said to have been born by falling in the form of a newborn serpent into the hands of his mother as she was offering water in worship of the sun. She called him Patanjali, from *pata,* meaning both "serpent" and "fallen," and *añjali,* referring to the gesture of her hands cupped in worship.[8] This story, like the story of Chudala, features a spiritually adept woman, both stories thus suggesting the Tantric dimensions of yoga. In Tantric practices, as in yoga, the norms of society are consciously overturned in order to liberate practitioners from their worldly constraints and release an explosion of energy that gives initiates extraordinary powers.

Patanjali did not invent yoga; it has its origins deep in India's past. The aphorisms of the *Yoga Sutra* text draw on various ancient traditions of yoga. The text also incorporates direct allusions to important philosophical and psychological ideas of ancient India, which create a foil for Patanjali's analyses.

Scholars hypothesize that some form of yoga may belong to the earliest periods of civilization on the Indian subcontinent, evidence for which comes from archaeological artifacts dating from the third millennium B.C. found in the Indus River valley. The still undeciphered written records are inscribed on seals that depict animal and human forms. Among these is a horned anthropomorphic figure surrounded by animals and seated in the cross-legged position that is a basic posture of yoga.

A suggestive reference to yoga is later found in the *Rig Veda,* the ancient collection of hymns associated with the Indo-European sacrificial cult and dating to about 1000 B.C.[9] One hymn describes ascetics with long, streaming hair who overcome the limitations of the body (RV 10.136).[10] Like the adepts discussed in the *Yoga Sutra,* they acquire enormous magical powers, such as the ability to travel through the air and know the thoughts of others.

In the middle of the first millennium B.C., Indian political and religious ferment spawned two enormous bodies of oral literature in which various forms of yoga are prominent: the teachings of the Buddha and the Hindu epic poems, the *Ramayana* and the *Mahabharata.* In both, yoga is defined in terms of discipline of the senses and mind that adepts practice in order to achieve access to the deeper recesses of spiritual insight and power.

The most ancient sustained expression of yogic ideas is found in the early sermons of the Buddha, who lived in the latter half of the sixth century B.C. His sermons are preserved in the oldest collection of Buddhist texts, known as the Pali Canon. Both the "Four Noble Truths" and the "Eightfold Path," articulated in the Buddha's first sermon in the Deer Park, contain elements that underlie the yoga system.[11] The *Yoga Sutra* was certainly composed much later, but the elements that it shares with Buddhism may come from a common store of contemplative practice that was incorporated into Buddhism and developed there.[12] The important role of Buddhist technical terminology and concepts in the *Yoga Sutra* suggests that Patanjali was aware of Buddhist ideas and wove them into his system.[13] Two striking examples are the use of the term *nirodha* in the opening definition of yoga as *citta-vṛtti-nirodha,* "cessation of the turnings of thought" (1.2), and the statement that "all is suffering (*duḥkha*) for the wise man" (2.15). *Duḥkha* and *nirodha* are crucial terms in the Buddhist doctrine of the Four Noble Truths, where they refer to the fact of universal suffering and to the means for the cessation of suffering, respectively.[14]

The doctrine of suffering is the core of what Buddhists believe to be the first sermon taught by the Buddha after he achieved enlightenment. In the long meditation that led up to his enlightenment, the Buddha realized that the transience of pleasure and of life itself is a constant source of sorrow, which is deepened by the human desire for permanence in a constantly changing world. He perceived that suffering could be stopped only through the complete cessation of craving. From the point of view of the Buddha and Patanjali alike, the suffering that is fundamental to the human condition is a defilement that can be removed through religious and meditative practice.

The psychology of both yoga and Buddhism focuses on freedom from worldly suffering through a liberating practice. Meditation and mental discipline in various forms are basic to the practice of Buddhism. The practical means to freedom has eight "limbs" in each system, of which six elements are common to both. The Buddha and Patanjali both prescribed moral behavior, control of the breath, control of the senses, celibacy, meditation, and pure contemplation (*samādhi*) that brings liberating insight into the true nature of things.[15]

During the same period that Buddhism was developing, a concern with yoga was expressed in early Indian epic literature.[16] In the *Mahabharata,* the vast Indian epic of war between enemy cousins—a war that ends in the annihilation of both armies—the warriors acquire their supernatural powers and weapons through physical discipline and meditative practices that are akin to the practices later codified by Patanjali.

In the *Mahabharata,* the most masterful practitioner of yoga is Arjuna, the exemplary warrior and disciple of the god Krishna. In more than one episode, Arjuna performs extraordinary feats of yogic austerity to enhance his mental and physical prowess. The most famous episode does not, however, involve physical action, but rather turns on Arjuna's participation in a mystical dialogue with Krishna. In this dialogue, known as the *Bhagavad Gita,* Krishna teaches Arjuna the varied forms of yogic discipline.[17] The battlefield setting of the *Gita* is not only a physical place, but a state of mind. As the war is about to begin, Arjuna's nerve fails at the thought of doing battle against his cousins and other family members. Krishna explains to him that it is a warrior's duty to kill: instead of shrinking from this duty, Arjuna must learn to renounce the selfish attachment to the fruits of his actions. Krishna teaches him to discipline his thought and emotion so that he can perform the necessary action, free from bloodlust and pain. The way to this goal is through physical and psychological discipline, concentration, meditation, and contemplative awareness.

Although Krishna's teaching agrees with that of Patanjali in emphasizing the primacy of detachment and mental discipline in gaining spiritual liberation, there are fundamental differences. In the *Gita* liberation enables one to wage the battle of life, while in the *Yoga Sutra* liberation entails an absolute isolation of the spirit from all worldly concerns. This liberation is impossible, however, without a commitment to the moral principles (*yama*) and observances (*niyama*) of the yoga system. The doctrine of the *Gita* vibrates with the imagery of mystical friendship, mental attitudes transformed through devotion, and action performed with spiritual skill and in an attitude of sacrifice. At the core of Patanjali's yoga, in contrast, is a total cessation of all mental activity and suspension of all physical action. While dedication to the Lord (*īśvara*) is referred to in the *Yoga Sutra* (1.24), *īśvara* is not a creator god. Patanjali does not furnish details, but the context suggests that he conceived the Lord as an eternal, archetypal yogi, an object of concentration for the practitioner who seeks to achieve spiritual calm. Nowhere in the *Yoga Sutra* is *īśvara* defined as an omnipotent god like Krishna in the *Gita,* who manifests himself as the Lord of Life and Death.

In the *Gita,* yoga is defined in various ways. In the second chapter, it is characterized as "equanimity" (2.48) and "skill in action" (2.50), a skill achieved only when understanding breaks through delusion and remains immovable in pure contemplation (*samādhi*). The practitioner is warned that if his mind becomes attached to the play of the senses, they can drive away insight, as wind drives a ship on water (2.67); rather, he must withdraw his senses, like a tortoise retracting its limbs (2.58).

Later in his teaching, Krishna describes the discipline of the yogi in terms that are even closer to the doctrine elaborated in the *Yoga Sutra.* In the sixth chapter of the *Gita,* Arjuna responds to Krishna's definition of yoga as equanimity (*sāmya*) by protesting that such a state is an impossibility, given the condition of the mind as faltering, violent, and stubborn—as difficult to hold as the wind (6.34). In the following verse Krishna responds in words that are echoed in the *Yoga Sutra,* saying that practice and dispassion can restrain the mind.

Throughout the *Mahabharata,* the practice of mental and physical discipline, referred to as yoga, is allied with a dualistic theory of cosmic evolution known as *sāṅkhya.* These practical and theoretical ideas develop separately outside the epic context, each becoming a distinct Hindu philosophical system with its own foundation text and exegetical tradition.[18] As these systems developed, Yoga philosophy became the field of practical philosophical analysis and meditative experimentation, while the Sankhya system emphasized the theoretical analysis of cosmic evolution.[19]

Hindu scholastic culture classifies orthodox philosophy into six systems, two of which are Yoga and Sankhya. In this classification, the philosophy and spiritual practice of the Yoga school—which has as its foundation text Patanjali's *Yoga Sutra*—is regarded as a complement to the theoretical cosmogony of Sankhya.[20] The Sankhya text parallel to the *Yoga Sutra* is the *Sankhya Karika,* attributed to Ishvara Krishna. It presents an abstract analysis of the constituents of phenomenal existence and the evolution of the universe out of primordial matter.[21] Yoga, as a code of practical discipline, is amplified by the Sankhya model of cosmic evolution, the psychological condition of the individual mirroring the Sankhya cosmogony in microcosm. The basis of spiritual liberation in the Yoga school is a profound experience of the evolutionary process whereby spirit becomes enmeshed in material nature.

Common to both systems is a universe structured in terms of two primal principles—spirit (*puruṣa*) and material nature (*prakṛti*). Both are extreme abstractions, like superstrings in modern cosmology. In its undifferentiated state, spirit is eternally inactive, while material nature evolves from within itself into the entire world of creation and destruction. The analysis presupposes an idealized state of cosmic equilibrium in which spirit exists in balance with, but isolated from, material nature. It is only when this equilibrium is disturbed that creation occurs.

Spirit (*puruṣa*) is an abstraction from the knowable world. Like a point in Euclidean geometry, spirit has no material identity except in relation to the phenomenal world. According to Patanjali, it is through ignorance that the spirit is connected to this world. Alone, it is pure consciousness, the ground of nonconceptual, spiritual knowledge.

According to the Sankhya system, all material nature (*prakṛti*) is composed of three distinct qualities (*guṇa*), which are like aspects of energy existing in potential form and actualized in innumerable combinations throughout the material world.[22] The qualities are lucidity (*sattva*), the pure, clear quality of nature's perfection; passion (*rajas*), the quality of energy and motivation; and dark inertia (*tamas*), which weighs down the other two. Among the twenty-four evolutes of primal matter enumerated in Sankhya theory, Patanjali's teaching focuses on those that must be understood in order to break open the gross and subtle fetters of thought. The relation that binds spirit to the material world is difficult to understand, since the very faculties of understanding are themselves material in nature—thought (*citta*), mind (*manas*), intelligence (*buddhi*), and ego (*ahaṃkāra*).[23]

The thought process (*citta*) is a combination of the other three psychomental evolutes of matter. Together with the five sense organs (*indriya*), this thought process is the means whereby individual cognition and emotion function. Unlike *manas,* which is the organ of thought and with which *citta* is often misidentified, *citta,* thought, encompasses the entire mental capacity. Being part of the material realm, thought is plastic and subject to various modifications, which Patanjali characterizes as the "turnings of thought" (*citta-vṛtti*). These turnings comprise all the states of consciousness. Patanjali regards thought in the phenomenal world as ceaselessly in motion, existing only in its modifications. The goal of yoga is to still this motion and so liberate the subject from the tyranny of uncontrollable thought.

Since mind is an aspect of material nature, mental tranquility is not in itself sufficient to ensure ultimate freedom—although one can begin to realize one's true humanity only when the mind is tranquil. But as long as the mind is muddled with wandering thoughts, it is impossible to discriminate between what is essential and what is adventitious.[24]

In Patanjali's view, the body and mind are physical and mental dimensions of the same material nature (*prakṛti*). However, interior nature—encompassing thought, mind, intelligence, and ego—is much more difficult to control than external nature. Physical forces are but gross manifestations of subtle mental forces. If the subtle, internal aspects of material nature are under control, control of the gross aspects is relatively easy—which accounts for the extraordinary powers a yogi can command.

In order to penetrate the logic of Patanjali's method, it seems crucial to grasp his analysis of how spirit (*puruṣa*) becomes bound to material nature (*prakṛti*) through the workings of thought (*citta*) and the accumulation of subliminal memory "traces" or "impressions" (*saṃskāra, vāsanā, āśaya*).

The central notion here is that any mental or physical act leaves behind memory "impressions" or "traces" that can subtly influence a person's thought, character, and moral behavior. The store of memory is composed of subliminal impressions (*saṃskāra*) and memory traces (*vāsanā*), which are the residue of experience that clings to an individual throughout life and, in the Indian view, from death to rebirth. The relation between the "turnings of thought" (*citta-vṛtti*) and memory is basic to Patanjali's epistemology. When thought passes from one modification into another, the former state is not lost but rather is preserved in memory as a subliminal impression or memory trace. Thus, thought is always generating memories, and these memories are a store of potential thoughts, available to be actualized into new turnings of thought. The very habit of thinking not only generates but preserves memories, like the roots of a tuber that spread underground and produce fresh tubers which blossom in season.

Memory is crucial to the production of religious and aesthetic experience throughout Sanskrit literature. In religious and literary texts there is a recurrent association between memory and the bondage of love.[25] The poets based their conception of memory on established philosophical notions. Indian epistemologists hold that whatever we perceive by means of the sense organs leaves an impression on the mind; memory occurs when a latent impression is awakened. Indian literary theorists accordingly define memory as a recollection of a condition of happiness or misery, whether it was conceived solely in the mind or actually occurred.

In what is considered one of the key passages of Sanskrit aesthetics, the tenth-century Kashmiri philosopher Abhinavagupta comments on what Kalidasa means by "memory" in his famous drama *Shakuntala.*[26] To illustrate Kalidasa's perspective Abhinavagupta cites the final verse from the opening scene of the fifth act of *Shakuntala,* in which the poet presents a compressed version of his aesthetic of memory. The king and the court buffoon are listening to a song being sung by Lady Hamsapadika, whom the king once loved but has since forgotten. The king muses to himself, "Why did hearing the song's words fill me with such strong desire? I'm not parted from anyone I love." The scene continues with this verse:

> Seeing rare beauty,
> hearing lovely sounds,
> even a happy man
> becomes
> strangely uneasy . . .
> perhaps he remembers,
> without knowing why,
> loves of another life
> buried deep in his being.

Memory, then, is not a discursive recollection of past events but rather an intuitive insight into the past that transcends personal experience, into the imaginative universe that beauty evokes.

In Patanjali's analysis, the aggregate of impressions that expresses itself in thought (*citta*) and action (*karma*) also accounts for subconscious predispositions that condition the character and behavior of an individual through many reincarnations. Thought and action thus become involved in an endless round of reciprocal causality. Actions create memory traces, which fuel the mental processes and are stored in memory, which endures through many rebirths. The store of subliminal impressions is obliterated only when the chain of causal relations is broken. But memory, reason, and even intuition have no relevance to the attainment of spiritual perfection and freedom. Liberation of the spirit is possible only when subconscious subliminal impressions are consumed and all the turnings of thought cease. In other words, the problem of freedom hinges on detachment from the perceived world of physical and mental activity. Such detachment loosens the bonds of memory that bind one to phenomenal existence, allowing one to realize the possibility of spiritual freedom.

Cultivation of mental tranquility is crucial to reversing the accumulation of psychological fetters, for only when thought is tranquil can one realize one's spiritual nature. A person whose mind is bewildered by wandering thoughts is caught in the web of those thoughts. Since thought is fundamental to the spirit's involvement with material nature, the way to extricate one's spirit is to make thought invulnerable to the chaos of mental and physical stimuli. In order to achieve such a state, one must perfect one's body and mind by conquering passionate attachment through the disciplined practice that Patanjali prescribes.

PATANJALI'S TEXT

The 195 aphorisms (*sūtra*s, literally "threads") that make up the *Yoga Sutra* outline a practical means for realizing spiritual perfection through distinct modes of discipline. In the aphorisms Patanjali seems to be refining a set of essential ideas drawn from a mass of varied material on the nature of mental discipline and spiritual freedom. Each aphorism distills in a single phrase some element of the complex "methodology" for radically rethinking one's relation to the world and revising one's perception of the entire structure of thought.

The *Yoga Sutra* is divided into four sections. The first deals with the cessation of thought and the cultivation of pure contemplation. The second explains the eight limbs of yogic practice and the systematic means to succeed in this practice, while the third is devoted to the last three of the limbs of this practice, an integrated discipline that gives the yogi extraordinary knowledge and powers. Finally, the fourth section explores the nature of absolute spiritual freedom, which is the ultimate goal of yoga.[27]

The first section of the text presents a set of definitions and establishes relations among the different modes of achieving mental tranquility and spiritual liberation. The entire text is informed by the opening definition of yoga as the "cessation of the turnings of thought," following which "the spirit stands in its true identity as observer to the world." Patanjali then elaborates the basic methods of bringing thought to stillness, a process that allows the self to be a pure observer (*draṣṭṛ*) in relation to the visible world of phenomenal experience, without participating in it. This section also introduces two major components of yogic practice—the cultivation of dispassion and dedication to the Lord (*īśvara*), the supreme spirit of yoga. Its main subject, however, is pure contemplation (*samādhi*), a spiritual integration that leads to absolute independence of the spirit from involvement with the material world. This independence is as paradoxical and difficult to describe as it is to attain, but those few who seem to have experienced it attest to a spiritual freedom beyond time and place.

The second section of the text presents the practical body of Patanjali's teaching, whose core is the eightfold discipline of yoga (*aṣṭāṅga-yoga*). Before going on to present details of the eightfold path, Patanjali analyzes the causes of the error and suffering that are obstacles to spiritual liberation. These forces of corruption are identified as ignorance, egoism, passion, hatred, and the will to live. Ignorance, which is the root of the other corruptions, is a misunderstanding of the interaction between the observing spirit (*puruṣa*) and the phenomenal world (*prakṛti*). It misleads us into egotistically believing in a unified self and falsely identifying spirit with matter.

Fortunately, ignorance can be eliminated by a serious commitment to living the disciplined life of a yogi. The practice of a dedicated yogi consists of eight interrelated disciplines of spiritual development that culminate in pure contemplation of one's inner truth. When ignorance is dispelled, the spirit exists as an observer to the world, free from attachment to the world's painful transience.

The third section is largely devoted to detailing the power one gains by perfecting the practice of yoga. The concentrated energy that accumulates through contemplation and spiritual control gives the yogi's thought a flexibility that allows it to transcend the constraints of ordinary knowledge and attain limitless powers. These powers manifest themselves to the yogi in the hyperconscious state of perfect discipline (*saṃyama*). The transformation that thought undergoes through concentration, meditation, and pure contemplation—the final three limbs of yogic practice, which constitute perfect discipline—enables thought to discriminate between material nature and the observing spirit. This opens one to the extraordinary powers of thought, such as knowledge of past and future, as well as of one's former births, knowledge of others' thoughts, supernormal hearing and sight, the ability to enter into other bodies, to become invisible, and to understand the different languages of humans, as well as those of animals and birds. In enumerating and describing these powers Patanjali gives us images of the mind's potential to achieve the seemingly impossible inward journey to spiritual freedom, a state beyond all boundaries and limits. Although the experience of these powers thus serves a definite purpose on the yogi's path, the temptation to succumb to their magical potency must be overcome if the yogi is to proceed toward freedom. It is as though the yogi must experience the full extent of the power of thought before being able to bring about its absolute cessation, which is the culmination of yogic practice.

This section of the *Yoga Sutra* echoes shamanic practice in some ways. However, the ultimate goal of yogic practice is not the attainment of magical powers and ecstatic states, but spiritual freedom. The emphasis placed on the shaman's instinctive ability to conjure the unseen world of gods, demons, and ancestral spirits is downplayed in yoga. The miraculous powers of the shaman are within the capacity of a yogi, but they are deemed dangerous in that they can distract one who possesses them from the goal of spiritual freedom.[28]

Few ancient Indian philosophers take the hyperbole surrounding these powers literally. Indian myth and literature, however, are filled with stories of yogis whose powers enable them to defy the laws of nature. Their powers threaten even the gods, who use various means of seduction to control the yogis. A striking example occurs in the story of Rishyashringa, a young ascetic born of a doe in the forest and trained in yoga by his father in total isolation from human society, including the pleasures of women.[29] When a drought devastates the land near the forest where Rishyashringa dwells, priests instruct the king to send wily courtesans to lure the boy to the capital in hopes of harnessing his yogic energy to relieve the drought. His innocence makes him susceptible to their enticements, and he is eventually overcome by the beauty of the king's nubile daughter. His yogic energy thus released, the rains fall. Although Rishyashringa lives on in the world as a great sage, from the viewpoint of the *Yoga Sutra,* his story illustrates how vulnerable even an advanced yogi is to the distractions of the world that his own increasing powers expose.

The warning about the powers of yoga is a prelude to the fourth section of the *Yoga Sutra,* where Patanjali examines the aspects of thought and action that constitute the final obstacles to absolute spiritual freedom (*kaivalya*). This section recapitulates ideas presented in earlier sections of the text from the perspective of the omniscient observer, who is able to realize the independence of the spirit from its involvement with material nature. For the independent spirit, liberation is not the extinction of individual existence, but a potent state of calm. In the course of his analysis of the relations among action, thought, memory, and liberating knowledge, Patanjali alludes to various ideas about causality, mainly drawn from more detailed Sankhya theories of cause and effect.[30]

In commenting on this section, Indian writers cite variants of the parable of the lost son to explain how the yogi comes to realize the true nature of the spirit. A king's son, born into court intrigue, is abandoned in infancy and reared by outcastes, with whom he identifies himself. Through the offices of an aged minister, however, he is found and told that he is now king, and not an outcaste at all. At first, he is unable to understand, but under the minister's careful tutelage, his self-perception is changed, and he gradually comprehends what it means to be king. Likewise, the yogi can come to realize the true state of his spirit by cultivating the discrimination that allows him to distinguish between the spirit as knowing observer and the phenomenal world of material nature.

THE STYLE OF THE TEXT

The *Yoga Sutra* is written in a simple, aphoristic style, which contrasts sharply with the rhetorical complexity of the commentaries. The language is spare and often extremely technical. There is a virtual absence of metaphors, and even similes are kept to a minimum. In the *Yoga Sutra,* the aim is not to make connections but to disengage the illusory connection between the spirit and nature. The minimalist aphorisms and absence of metaphor underscore Patanjali's central point that one must transcend all relational thinking in order to realize the isolation of absolute freedom.

Although the commentators have not taken sufficient note of this, the text has an internal structure and coherence that abounds with cross-references. Each aphorism contributes to the whole, even though the interpretation of an individual aphorism often depends on the specific philosophical context in which Patanjali is making his point.

The terse, elliptical nature of the aphorisms has attracted varying interpretations of both the whole and its parts. The earliest surviving commentary is the *Yogabhashya* of Vyasa (eighth century A.D.), which is itself the subject of a study called the *Tattvavaisharadi* by Vacaspati Mishra (ninth century). Both have been translated into English, and one of the most reliable translations of them remains the 1914 version of J. H. Woods.[31] The Vyasa commentary, which belongs to the early Indian scholastic tradition, is concerned with the philosophical meaning of the aphorisms. It was Vyasa who established the main interpretive tradition relating to the text, a tradition still followed by the majority of Indian and Western interpreters and translators. Subsequent commentaries amplify details of yogic practice that Patanjali only alludes to. As is the case with other aphoristic foundation texts, the *Yoga Sutra* has gained much of its authority within the tradition of Hindu philosophy by the weight of commentarial material attached to it, and the scores of interpretations undeniably aid us in penetrating the layers of meaning embedded in the text. At the same time, though, they often obscure Patanjali's elegant critique of the mental attitudes that bind us to suffering the vagaries of material existence.

A recently discovered, and controversial, subcommentary on Vyasa's commentary has been attributed to the great philosopher of the monistic Vedanta school, Shankara, who lived in the ninth century. Even if the attribution of the commentary is inauthentic, it does attest to the interest shown by Vedanta scholars in the philosophical implications of Patanjali's ideas. As in later Vedantic interpretations, there is an emphasis on a transcendent dimension to yoga that is absent in Patanjali's philosophy of cessation and spiritual liberation. It is in fact difficult to reconcile the antimetaphorical stance of the *Yoga Sutra* with the ancient Vedantic idea—prevalent in the late Vedic hymns and the *Upanishads*—that if one discovers correspondences between apparently dissimilar things, one can understand the essence of the cosmos. Patanjali presents an incisive, radical philosophical analysis of mental discipline that seems blunted by Vedantic ideas.

Indeed, it is the radicalism of Patanjali's analysis that makes the *Yoga Sutra* so compelling. In my view, even if one cannot completely follow the system that Patanjali outlines or pursue the discipline to its fulfillment, the style and structure of the text communicate its strategy with a directness that renders it comprehensible to a dedicated reader. In a very important sense, the act of becoming aware of these issues constitutes a step on the way.

Granted, it is unlikely that any uninitiated reader can fully understand a text whose interpretation has been debated for centuries by scholars and practitioners, both Indian and Western. Within Indian tradition, the *Yoga Sutra* is an economical set of mnemonic pronouncements on the arduous course for achieving spiritual freedom, a text that is meant to be learned by heart and amplified by a teacher's guidance, although ultimately it can only be fully apprehended experientially, through long, continuous practice. Still, if one approaches a reading of the aphorisms as a kind of experiment, there is much to be gained. Even if one is unable to understand all the details of the analysis, one can explore Patanjali's philosophical and psychological terrain—like a traveler in a strange country, exploring a new landscape and absorbing its contours before observing its details. The text can be understood on various levels of sophistication, but the core of Patanjali's worldview is apparent to any reader who will make the effort.

The goal of yogic transformation is realized in contemplative practice. The path to freedom consists of a gradual unwinding of misconceptions that allows for fresh perceptions. It is as if one were walking attentively through a forest in which one could not precisely identify every animal, bird, flower, and tree. Even so, the sounds of the various creatures, the smells of flowers and ferns, and the shapes of trees move one toward a more acute awareness of the environment, and in this process of reorientation the contours of the landscape change. The way of yoga is not a simple, linear path. Rather, it is a complex method involving a radical change in the way we experience the world and conceive the process of knowing ourselves. It gives us techniques with which to analyze our own thought processes and finally to lay bare our true human identity.

Yoga

Discipline of Freedom

PART ONE

Cessation of Thought and Contemplative Calm

THE NATURE OF YOGA

This is the teaching of yoga. (1)
Yoga is the cessation of the turnings of thought. (2)
When thought ceases, the spirit stands in its true identity as observer to the world. (3)
Otherwise, the observer identifies with the turnings of thought. (4)

The first four aphorisms define the nature of yoga as a state of mental tranquility and spiritual freedom, as well as the means to achieve this state. These aphorisms also introduce technical terms that will recur and be elaborated throughout the text as Patanjali clarifies his view of human psychology. In the self-reflexive style characteristic of Indian philosophical texts, the *Yoga Sutra* contains various complementary definitions of yoga. This first definition establishes the focus of the doctrine.

Yoga is defined as *citta-vṛtti-nirodha,* "cessation of the turnings of thought." The text will be concerned throughout with *citta,* which may be translated as "thought"—the sensitive, subtle aspects of the mental capacity.[1] Thought exists in the form of its activity, or "turning" (*vṛtti*). "The turnings of thought" (*citta-vṛtti*) refers to the totality of mental processes—conscious, subconscious, and hyperconscious—not simply to the faculties of intellect, recollection, or emotion. Although *citta* is often translated as "mind," this blurs the contrast with *manas. Manas* is the organ of cognition, whereas *citta* is the total process of thought. This thought process is a composite of mind (*manas*), intelligence (*buddhi*), and ego (*ahaṃkāra*), the three mental evolutes of material nature (*prakṛti*).

Thus, in Patanjali's view, thought is fundamental to the spirit's involvement with material nature. The way to extricate one's spirit is by making thought invulnerable to stimulation by the world of experience. "Cessation" (*nirodha*) means that the turnings of thought have stopped.

Insofar as the subtle mental processes are active, the subject or self is necessarily unstable and agitated. The goal of yoga is to stop the thought processes so that the spirit can be free, isolated from the turmoil of thought from which it mistakenly takes its identity. This idea is echoed in the *Bhagavad Gita,* where Krishna says of the yogi: "He should gradually become tranquil, firmly controlling his understanding; focusing his mind on the self, he should think nothing" (6.25).

The observer (*draṣṭṛ*) is the subject who watches the visible world of phenomenal experience but who does not participate in it. For the observer everything extrinsic to itself—even the subtleties of thought—is witnessed with detachment, rather than experienced. "Observer" is also a designation for the spirit (*puruṣa*) in its conscious aspect (cf. 2.12, 20).

THE TURNINGS OF THOUGHT

> The turnings of thought, whether corrupted or immune to the forces of corruption, are of five kinds. (5)
> They are valid judgment, error, conceptualization, sleep, and memory. (6)
> The valid means of judgment are direct perception, inference, and verbal testimony. (7)
> Error is false knowledge with no objective basis. (8)
> Conceptualization comes from words devoid of substance. (9)
> Sleep is the turning of thought abstracted from existence. (10)
> Memory is the recollection of objects one has experienced. (11)

Patanjali delineates five modes of thought, each of which can be either corrupted or immune to corruption. The nature of "corruption" will be defined at greater length in Part Two (see 2.4–9), but it is important to note here that even the most subtle and benign workings of thought are obstructions to freedom of the spirit.

Valid judgment is based on one of the three legitimate methods for accurately apprehending material reality (7). Error is false knowledge that has no such basis in fact. Conceptualization is the tendency of thought to construct an image of reality that has no foundation beyond individual subjectivity. We may thus have verbal knowledge in which words and meanings fail to correspond to any objective reality.

Sleep includes both dreaming and dreamless states. "Thought abstracted from existence" is a liberal rendering of *abhāvapratyayālambanā,* which more literally means "founded on the awareness of nonexistence."[2]

Memory is basic to Patanjali's epistemology. No thought is ever lost; rather, it is preserved as a subliminal impression or memory trace. These traces not only allow us to recall past events and perceptions, but they also actively shape future experiences in a never-ending process.

PRACTICE AND DISPASSION

> Cessation of the turnings of thought comes through practice and dispassion. (12)
> Practice is the effort to maintain the cessation of thought. (13)
> This practice is firmly grounded when it is performed for a long time without interruption and with zeal. (14)
> Dispassion is the sign of mastery over the craving for sensuous objects. (15)
> Higher dispassion is a total absence of craving for anything material, which comes by discriminating between spirit and material nature. (16)

Patanjali now turns to the question of how thought may be stilled. Aphorisms 12 through 40 describe the many paths to this single goal. All involve some form of practice leading to dispassion.

Yogic practice is the link between the ordinary self and ultimate freedom of spirit. In Patanjali's philosophy, we are not dependent on any external agency to grant us this freedom. It is achieved over time through our own efforts and through discipline. Practitioners may progress slowly or quickly, and may achieve different degrees of detachment or dispassion. These differences will be discussed in subsequent aphorisms.

A recognition, however tentative, that the spirit is distinct from material nature makes the practitioner disinterested in material things—even those which seem desirable or good. This detachment from material desire is an important step toward spiritual freedom. It culminates in Patanjali's "higher dispassion"—a complete detachment from the world of experience, in which we cease to identify ourselves with the material world.

WAYS OF STOPPING THOUGHT

Conscious cessation of thought can arise from various forms of conjecture, reflection, enjoyment, and egoism. (17)

Beyond this is a state where only subliminal impressions remain from the practice of stopping thought. (18)

For gods and men unencumbered by physical bodies, but still enmeshed in material nature, the cessation of thought is limited by reliance on the phenomenal world. (19)

> For others cessation of thought follows from faith, heroic energy, mindfulness, contemplative calm, and wisdom. (20)
> For those who possess a sharp intensity, it is immediate. (21)
> Higher than this is cessation beyond distinctions of mild, moderate, or extreme. (22)

The meaning of this crucial section has been controversial since ancient times. Most commentators say that these aphorisms refer to levels of contemplative calm (*samādhi*). Others, however, argue that they refer to the cessation of thought (*nirodha*), and this is the interpretation I develop here. All of Part One of the *Yoga Sutra* seems to explore the meaning and means of bringing thought to rest; contemplative calm is given as just one of the states that can lead to cessation of thought (20).

According to Patanjali, the cessation of the turnings of thought comes about in various ways. On the first level, ordinary conscious processes are directed toward the aim of stilling thought's activity (17). On subsequent levels, cessation involves hyperconscious processes in which every modification of thought is eliminated and only the subliminal impressions of past experience remain. The conscious restraint of thought is related to the seeded contemplation of 1.46.

The subliminal impressions (*saṃskāra*) are the residue left on the mind by past thoughts, actions, and reactions to sense stimuli. These are forgotten and lie latent in the subconscious mind, eventually to ripen and set up new mental processes—lasting even from one incarnation to the next. In order to quiet the thought processes completely, one would have to clear the mind of all impressions. But this is extremely difficult, so Patanjali offers various ways of controlling their formation and using their power.[3]

Here the distinction between conscious and hyperconscious modes of cessation is supplemented by reference to other modes, probably drawn from various contemporaneous theories of how to achieve spiritual freedom. Aphorism 19 discusses figures from Indian myth, gods and heroes who are free from the ordinary constraints of their physical bodies but whose mental condition and store of impressions from previous lives keep them attached to material nature.

The fivefold power of faith, heroic energy, mindfulness, contemplative calm, and wisdom parallels identical aspects of early Buddhist practice.[4] Patanjali clearly shares the Buddhist view that right living and a long process of spiritual cultivation have the power to effect extraordinary mental transformations. These practices are then contrasted with the higher forms of mental exercise that Patanjali is about to reveal, forms in which the subliminal impressions instantly vanish and all thought ceases.

DEDICATION TO THE LORD OF YOGA

Cessation of thought may also come from dedication to the Lord of Yoga. (23)

The Lord of Yoga is a distinct form of spirit unaffected by the forces of corruption, by actions, by the fruits of action, or by subliminal intentions. (24)

In the Lord of Yoga is the incomparable seed of
omniscience. (25)
Being unconditioned by time, he is the teacher of even
the ancient teachers. (26)
His sound is the reverberating syllable *AUM.* (27)
Repetition of this syllable reveals its meaning. (28)

The identification and role of the Lord (*īśvara*) in yoga varies according to schools of practice and philosophical interpretation. For Patanjali, the Lord is not a creator god who grants grace; rather, he is a representation of the omniscient spirit (*puruṣa*) as the archetypal yogi (*yogeśvara*). The definition of *īśvara* as "a distinct form of the spirit" (*puruṣa*) (24) identifies it with the primary spiritual principle of Sankhya.

"Lord of Yoga" is a common epithet of the Hindu ascetic-god Shiva. In the *Bhagavad Gita,* the warrior-god Krishna is also called *yogeśvara,* the embodiment of the yogic practice he teaches to his disciple Arjuna. In his teaching, Krishna refers to himself as "every creature's timeless seed."[5] Patanjali seems to be saying that the seed-cognition does not germinate in the Lord of Yoga, since he is self-contained and omniscient. This would also be the case for a yogi who has realized the true nature of his spirit.

Patanjali's use of the term dedication (*praṇidhāna*) (23) may be related to the Buddhist *bodhisattva praṇidhāna,* a vow to forgo final liberation (*nirvāṇa*) in order to help all other creatures attain enlightenment. This suggests that Patanjali's sense of dedication is not primarily one of worship, but rather one of commitment to the discipline represented by the Lord of Yoga.

Nonetheless, it also opens the way to synthesizing yogic practice with other religious and moral observances.

AUM is the primordial sound (*praṇava*), the cosmic vibration. Human beings may reproduce it by extending and strengthening the open compound vowel sound *AU* with the nasal sound *M*. The *AU* is generated deep in the body and is brought out through the nasal *M*, which then resonates in the head. According to the ancient Indian traditions preserved in the *Upanishads*, all speech and thought are derived from the one sound *AUM*. It expresses ultimate reality—in the cosmos, in the Lord of Yoga, and in the individual.[6]

OVERCOMING OBSTACLES AND DISTRACTIONS

> When *AUM* reveals itself, introspection is attained and obstacles fall away. (29)
>
> The obstacles that distract thought are disease, apathy, doubt, carelessness, indolence, dissipation, false vision, failure to attain a firm basis in yoga, and restlessness. (30)
>
> These distractions are accompanied by suffering, frustration, trembling of the body, and irregular breathing. (31)
>
> The practice of focusing on the single truth is the means to prevent these distractions. (32)

Patanjali pauses in his exploration of the paths to the cessation of thought in order to consider the obstacles that lie in the way. Before thought can cease entirely, the practitioner must withdraw from the phenomenal world and turn inward, attaining introspection. A host of distractions, however, both mental and physical, may arise to prevent this inner calm. Chanting the resonant syllable *AUM* clears away obstacles; this practice focuses the mind on "the single truth," the nature of the one reality (*tattva*).

TRANQUILITY OF THOUGHT

> Tranquility of thought comes through the cultivation of friendship, compassion, joy, and impartiality in spheres of pleasure or pain, virtue or vice. (33)
> Or through the measured exhalation and retention of breath. (34)
> Or when the mind's activity, arisen in the sense world, is held still. (35)
> Or when thought is luminous, free from sorrow. (36)
> Or when thought is without passion in the sphere of the senses. (37)
> Or when its foundation is knowledge from dreams and sleep. (38)
> Or through meditation on a suitable object. (39)
> For one whose thought is tranquil, mastery extends from the most minute particle to the vast expanse. (40)

In these aphorisms, Patanjali again offers a number of practices that lead to the preliminary goal of calming the thought processes.

The cultivation of friendship, compassion, joy, and impartiality echoes ancient practices followed by Buddhist monks to effect a radical change in their perceived relationship with other creatures on earth. These practices work to demolish the boundaries between oneself and others, and to break through the barriers that lock people into egoism. In Buddhist terms these practices bring about a transmutation of personal emotions into immeasurable virtues. Through impartiality toward all living beings—oneself, friends, strangers, enemies—the emotions of love, compassion, and joy are stabilized and universalized, enduring under any circumstances.[7]

The remaining aphorisms recapitulate practices that Patanjali has already described, and introduce others that will be further delineated in Part Two, including the yogic practice of breath control (*prāṇāyāma*) (34). Thought becomes luminous when it is freed from sorrow and passion, which are conceived of as heavy, dark, and opaque.

Thought may also be brought to tranquility through the knowledge gained in the deeper states of consciousness achieved in both dreams and dreamless sleep. These states are considered separate from—but not inferior to—waking reality. As Patanjali has said, they are "abstracted from existence" (1.10).

Aphorism 40 is the first description of the powers that result from yogic practice, which will be explored more fully in Part Three. Here, they are simply declared to encompass all of reality, from the microcosm to the macrocosm.

CONTEMPLATION THAT BEARS SEEDS

When the turnings of thought stop, a contemplative
poise occurs, in which thought, like a polished crystal, is

colored by what is nearby—whether perceiver, process of perception, or object of perception. (41)
When concepts formed from knowledge based on words and their meanings taint it, contemplative poise is broken by conjecture. (42)
When memory is purified, then contemplative poise is free of conjecture, empty of its own identity, with the object alone shining forth. (43)
Contemplative poise that is both reflective and intuitive, with subtle elements as its objects, is explained by this. (44)
The subtlety of objects results in their being free of defining marks. (45)
These modes of contemplative poise are the contemplation that bears seeds. (46)

This section deals with a technical aspect of the meditative process known as "contemplative poise" (*samāpatti*).[8] Here Patanjali uses one of his rare figures of speech to suggest how thought can become one with the object of thought. The yogi in whom the turnings of thought have ceased recognizes that thought, thus purified, is really colorless. But like a flawless crystal, it reflects, without distortion, the color of any object presented to it. This crystal-like thought allows for the realization of the nature of knowledge. It may take as its object any of the three components of knowledge: the knower or subject, the act of apprehension, or the object of perception—either singly or together.

The modes of *samāpatti* result from the various ways in which thought is modified into the form of the object. In the conjectural mode (42), thought focuses on the name and meaning of the object presented to it. In the nonconjectural mode (43), the preconceived names and identities of the object are eliminated as memory is cleansed. The distinction between knower, process of perception, and object dissolves.

Contemplative poise is pure when the fictions of verbal convention and inferential knowledge fall away. Then thought, without any conscious effort to know, is pervaded by the nature of the object of meditation.

Both the conjectural and nonconjectural modes of contemplative poise operate in the realm of sense organs and objects. Further refinement of the process involves what Patanjali terms the "subtle elements" (44). These have no recognizable name and form and give thought nothing to fix on, further disengaging it from the phenomenal world.

This analysis reflects Sankhya philosophical views, in which material nature evolves into gross and subtle elements. The gross elements are earth, air, fire, water, and space. Elements of the subtle sphere include ego, intelligence, mind, and the organs of sound, touch, shape, taste, and smell. Each of the gross elements is associated with a sense organ: thus air is related to sound and the ear; fire to sight and the eye; and so forth.[9] The difference between subtle and gross elements is that subtle elements are nonspecific and universal ("free of defining marks"), whereas gross elements are specific and particular.

Intuitive cognition (*nirvicāra*) (44) derives from the realization that the subjective world of spirit erroneously identifies itself with characteristics of material nature. This realization is suprarational, since the rational faculties of intelligence (*buddhi*) and mind (*manas*) belong to material nature.

Yet, insofar as thought depends on any object, however subtle, or even on a single idea, it is limited (46). In Patanjali's terms it has "seeds." Seed-bearing contemplation (*sabīja-samādhi*) is related to the conscious cessation of thought that leaves traces (1.17) and thus depends on subliminal impressions. Cognitive processes like conjecture, reflection, enjoyment, and egocentric perception are based on past experiences. If the pure tranquility of yoga is to be reached, these experiences must cease to develop into new experiences.

TOWARD SEEDLESS CONTEMPLATION

> The profound clarity of intuitive cognition brings inner tranquility. (47)
> Here wisdom is the vehicle of truth. (48)
> It has a different scope than scriptural or inferential knowledge because its object is singular. (49)
> A subliminal impression generated by wisdom stops the formation of other impressions. (50)
> When the turnings of thought cease completely, even wisdom ceases, and contemplation bears no seeds. (51)

In seed-bearing contemplation, the knowledge that spirit and material nature are fundamentally distinct is acquired through rational and intuitive means, which depend on memory. Contemplation without seeds (*nirbīja-samādhi*) is a hyperconscious condition in which thought is calm and totally integrated, so that it leaves no seeds to mature into further thoughts. This state of consciousness is a wisdom realized without intellectual activity.

Patanjali here contrasts this wisdom with the teachings of sacred texts and knowledge based on experience, which are fundamentally discursive and generate further thought. The extraordinary nature of this wisdom allows thought to flow while blocking the formation of new impressions—finally rendering itself superfluous in an absolute cessation of thought. Past experiences recorded in memory, reason, and even intuition have no relevance to the realization of the state of pure contemplation. Even the subliminal impressions that remain are consumed, and all turnings of thought cease.

PART TWO

The Practice of Yoga

THE PURPOSE OF YOGA

The active performance of yoga involves ascetic practice, study of sacred lore, and dedication to the Lord of Yoga. (1)

Its purpose is to cultivate pure contemplation and attenuate the forces of corruption. (2)

The forces of corruption are ignorance, egoism, passion, hatred, and the will to live. (3)

Patanjali now turns from defining the nature of yoga to the practical core of his teaching. The active performance of yoga, known as *kriyā-yoga,* is a threefold discipline involving ascetic practice, the study and chanting of sacred hymns and syllables, and dedication to the Lord of Yoga. These three elements constitute a subset of the second limb, called "observances" (*niyama*), of Patanjali's eight limbs of yoga, the path to spiritual liberation, which will be described in detail below. Although some commentators regard the active performance of yoga (*kriyā-yoga*) as referring collectively to the first five limbs of yogic practice, rather than to the observances alone, Patanjali's text itself clearly makes these three elements of *kriyā-yoga* a subset of the observances (see 2.32). These three practices are highlighted here to emphasize their particular efficacy in preparing the novice yogi for the arduous discipline that leads to pure contemplation by diminishing the forces that obstruct the path.

The forces of corruption (*kleśa*), which Patanjali will elaborate in the aphorisms that follow (2.4–9), arise out of our contact with the chaos of phenomenal existence and motivate our action in the world. Only by distancing ourselves from this mental and physical chaos through the practice of *kriyā-yoga* can the power of the corruptions be diminished.

Patanjali has already defined the Lord of Yoga as a form of spirit that is the omniscient teacher of the most ancient teachers and is unaffected by the corruptions (1.24–26). The divine yogi is a model for the practitioner who strives to eliminate the corrupting forces that make life painful.

DEFINITION OF THE FORCES OF CORRUPTION

Ignorance is the field where the other forces of
corruption develop, whether dormant, attenuated,
intermittent, or active. (4)

Ignorance is misperceiving permanence in transience,
purity in impurity, pleasure in suffering, an essential self
where there is no self. (5)

> Egoism is ascribing a unified self to the organs and powers of perception, such as the eye and the power to see. (6)
> Passion follows from attachment to pleasure. (7)
> Hatred follows from attachment to suffering. (8)
> The will to live is instinctive and overwhelming, even for a learned sage. (9)

Patanjali's notion of ignorance (*avidyā*) as the basic force of corruption reflects ancient Indian ideas about the root cause of suffering in the endless cycles of death and rebirth that constitute phenomenal existence. In the *Upanishads* ignorance is compared to a veil of illusion that covers the truth and confuses the mind so that it cannot discriminate between reality and appearance. In Buddhist analysis, ignorance is one of the twelve links in the causal chain of existence (*pratītyasamutpāda*).[10] Buddhists view the fundamental source of suffering as the false belief in an enduring individual self and the craving for permanence in a universe of impermanence.

For Patanjali ignorance is the basis of the other corrupting forces: egoism (*asmitā*), passion (*rāga*), hatred (*dveṣa*), and the will to live (*abhiniveśa*). Egoism is a false sense of self that comes about when we misidentify our essential nature with the material world. Passion and hatred flourish when we mistakenly define ourselves in terms of past pleasures and miseries, so that attachment to our memories of these experiences produces in us extreme feelings of desire or malice. The instinctual will to live is sustained by our attachment to life. This is so powerful that it afflicts even those who intellectually understand the transience of all things—unless they become disciplined in yoga.

REMOVING THE FORCES OF CORRUPTION

> The subtle forces of corruption can be escaped by reversing their course. (10)
> One can escape the effect of their turnings through meditation. (11)
> Subliminal intention formed in actions, rooted in the forces of corruption, is realized in present or potential births. (12)
> As long as this root exists, actions ripen into birth, a term of life, and experience in the world. (13)
> These actions bear joyful or sorrowful fruits according to the actor's virtue or vice. (14)
> All life is suffering for a man of discrimination, because of the sufferings inherent in change and its corrupting subliminal impressions, and because of the way qualities of material nature turn against themselves. (15)
> Suffering that has not yet come can be escaped. (16)

Patanjali now calls on Sankhya philosophy to explain how evolution is the transformation of primary, undifferentiated material nature (*prakṛti*) into the constituents of existence, such as egoism, mind, reason, the senses, and the subtle and gross elements. "Reversing the course" of the subtle forces of corruption is a kind of involution, the opposite of the evolutionary process. Patanjali seems to delineate three stages for the elimination of the corruptions: first they are diminished through *kriyā-yoga,* then their effects are avoided through meditation (*dhyāna*), but their total disappearance occurs only with the cessation of thought.

According to Patanjali, subliminal intentions (*āśaya*) bear fruit both in our current lifetime and in potential rebirths (*dṛṣṭādṛṣṭa-janma-vedanīya*). Forces of corruption create a ground on which impressions of the world take hold to form subliminal intentions. The commentator Vyasa suggests that a virtuous stock of such intentions results in rebirth as a god, while an evil stock results in a lower birth, as an insect, animal, or social outcast, for example. In Patanjali's analysis, the aggregate of impressions expresses itself in thought (*citta*) and action (*karma*), which account for subconscious predispositions that condition the character and behavior of an individual throughout many reincarnations. Thought and action then become involved in an endless round of reciprocal causality. Actions create memory traces, which fuel the mental processes and are stored in memory that endures through many rebirths. The store of subliminal impressions is obliterated only when the chain of causal relations is broken.

When the fruits of action (*karma*) and the seeds of thought are eliminated by means of meditation, thought no longer sustains the world, and what has evolved collapses into itself, like a black hole. The turnings (*vṛtti*) of the subtle forces of corruption can be eliminated, not by physical means, but through meditative insight, which cleans out the stock of invisible seeds that would otherwise germinate into new thoughts and actions.

The discriminating person knows that suffering is inherent in change, in the anxiety over change, and in the subliminal impressions left by this anxiety. The past and present are intertwined, and even pleasant experiences are tinged with pain. Suffering that is yet to come can be avoided, however, by relinquishing attachment to any desired outcome in the future, since such outcomes are illusory. Thus one eliminates the potential for suffering stored in subliminal impressions.

This section on the forces of corruption exhibits similarities with Buddhist discussions of methods by which defilements (*kleśa*) can be removed to eliminate suffering. Even though psychological modeling is crucial in both the yogic and Buddhist analyses, the objective is not merely a psychological shift but the actual removal of concrete defilements. This is the purificatory dimension of both yogic and Buddhist practice.

THE OBSERVER AND THE PHENOMENAL WORLD

The cause of suffering, which can be escaped, is the
connection between the observer and the phenomenal
world. (17)
The phenomenal world consists of material elements
and sense organs characterized by their clarity, activity,
or stillness; this world can serve the goals of sensual
experience or spiritual liberation. (18)
The qualities of material things are structured as
specific, nonspecific, marked, and unmarked. (19)
The observer is simply the subject of observing—
although pure, it sees itself in terms of conceptual
categories. (20)

In its essence the phenomenal world exists only in relation to an observer. (21)
Even if the phenomenal world ceases to be relevant for an observer who has realized freedom, it continues to exist because it is common to other observers. (22)
The connection between the observer and the phenomenal world causes a misperceived identity between active power and its master. (23)
The cause of this connection is ignorance. (24)
When there is no ignorance, there is no such connection—the freedom of the observer lies in its absence. (25)
The way to eliminate ignorance is through steady, focused discrimination between the observer and the world. (26)
Wisdom is the final stage of the sevenfold way of the observer. (27)

In these aphorisms, Patanjali analyzes the misunderstanding that binds the observing spirit (*puruṣa,* also called "the observer," *draṣṭṛ,* as at 1.3) to the phenomenal world (*prakṛti*). Ignorance of the true nature of this relation misleads us into egoistically believing in a unified self and falsely identifying spirit with matter. Since worldly existence occurs in an environment of corruptive forces, the unliberated spirit tends to be attracted by the phenomenal world, and misidentifies itself with it. This misidentification, together with the attachment to that misidentification, is the source of pain—but the connection can be severed by discrimination, which comes about through the practice of yoga. When ignorance is dispelled, the spirit becomes an observer to the world, detached from the world's painful transience (cf. 1.34; 2.6).

In order to effect this detachment, the yogi must understand the multidimensional structure of the world, in which everything is composed of the three qualities of material nature (*guṇa*). These qualities—lucidity (*sattva*), passion (*rajas*), and dark inertia (*tamas*)—are like energy existing in potential form. Among them, Patanjali is mainly concerned with lucidity, which he contrasts with spirit (see 3.35, 49, 55).

The qualities of material nature are structured into gross elements that can be particular or specific, subtle elements that can be universal or nonspecific, subtle matter that is differentiated or marked, and gross matter that is undifferentiated or unmarked. The misidentification of the power to act in the world (*śakti*) with its master, the spirit (*puruṣa*), is brought about by the false attribution of the qualities of material nature to the nature of the spirit itself.

The reference to a "sevenfold way" is somewhat obscure, since Patanjali does not elaborate on it. Commentators have proposed several versions of the sevenfold way and how its stages relate to the eight limbs of yogic practice described in the following sections.

THE LIMBS OF YOGIC PRACTICE

When impurity is destroyed by practicing the limbs of
yoga, the light of knowledge shines in focused
discrimination. (28)

> The eight limbs of yoga are moral principles, observances, posture, breath control, withdrawal of the senses, concentration, meditation, and pure contemplation. (29)

Patanjali's eight-limbed practice includes moral principles (*yama*), observances (*niyama*), posture (*āsana*), breath control (*prāṇāyāma*), withdrawal of the senses (*pratyāhāra*), concentration (*dhāraṇā*), meditation (*dhyāna*), and pure contemplation (*samādhi*). The eight limbs are essentially eight stages in the cumulative acquisition of yogic power. The first five will be elaborated in the remaining aphorisms of Part Two and the last three, which constitute the final stage of yoga, will be addressed in Part Three.

Patanjali's set of practices is parallel to the eight-limbed path of early Buddhism. In both yoga and Buddhism, this set of practices is crucial to the realization of spiritual freedom. The Buddhist eight-limbed path comprises right views, right speech, right conduct, right livelihood, right effort, right mindfulness, and right contemplation. Several of these are also central elements in Patanjali's practice: right conduct encompasses moral principles and observances, right mindfulness includes breath control and withdrawal of the senses, and right contemplation is equivalent to pure contemplation (*samādhi*).

THE MORAL PRINCIPLES AND OBSERVANCES

> The moral principles are nonviolence, truthfulness, abjuration of stealing, celibacy, and absence of greed. (30)

> These universal moral principles, unrestricted by conditions of birth, place, time, or circumstance, are the great vow of yoga. (31)
>
> The observances are bodily purification, contentment, ascetic practice, study of sacred lore, and dedication to the Lord of Yoga. (32)
>
> When one is plagued by ideas that pervert the moral principles and observances, one can counter them by cultivating the opposite. (33)
>
> Cultivating the opposite is realizing that perverse ideas, such as the idea of violence, result in endless suffering and ignorance—whether the ideas are acted out, instigated, or sanctioned, whether motivated by greed, anger, or delusion, whether mild, moderate, or extreme. (34)

A commitment to live according to the five universal moral principles (*yama*), without restrictions, constitutes the great vow (*mahāvrata*), which is the first step in undertaking yogic practice.[11] In distinct contrast to the relativity of values that characterizes caste Hinduism, where moral obligations and relations are relative to one's birth, for Patanjali social status is irrelevant to moral behavior.

Basic to Indian religious practice are vows of various kinds, such as the solemn vows to fast, to practice celibacy, and to perform acts of merit. The great vow of yoga parallels vows made by initiates in various Asian and Western ascetic traditions. Once the vow is made, the yogi proceeds to establish personal discipline through the observances (*niyama*) of bodily purification, contentment, austerity, study, and dedication to the Lord of Yoga.

The practice of "cultivating the opposite" involves recognizing that failure to follow the moral principles and observances leads to great pain and suffering throughout the world. For example, the opposite of nonviolence (*ahiṃsā*) is violence, which is destructive on both personal and universal levels. Violence not only harms the injured, but also the perpetrator of the violent act, who falls into an endless moral abyss. Any act of violence also increases the general level of destructive immorality in the world, while the practice of nonviolence increases the general good.

THE MORAL PRINCIPLES

> When one perseveres in nonviolence, hostility vanishes in its presence. (35)
> When one abides in truthfulness, activity and its fruition are grounded in the truth. (36)
> When one abjures stealing, jewels shower down. (37)
> When one observes celibacy, heroic energy accrues. (38)
> When one is without greed, the riddle of rebirth is revealed. (39)

Here, as with the observances that follow, Patanjali attributes direct results to specific moral actions, in a kind of reciprocal magic between the yogi and the world. The yogi's power of nonviolence is such that it neutralizes enmity in his presence.

Likewise, truthfulness assures the purity of actions and their fruit.[12]

According to Patanjali, the effects of the related moral principles of abjuring both stealing and greed are no less dramatic. He claims that if one renounces the attractions of the sensuous world that tempt one to covet and rob the wealth of others, real treasures accrue—"jewels" of inherent value and knowledge of the mystery of the cycles of birth and rebirth in transmigration.

THE OBSERVANCES

> Aversion to one's own body and avoidance of contact
> with others comes from bodily purification. (40)
> Also purity of intelligence, mental satisfaction, psychic
> focus, victory over the sense organs, and a vision of one's
> inner being. (41)
> Perfect happiness is attained through
> contentment. (42)
> Perfection of the body and senses comes from ascetic
> practice, which destroys impurities. (43)
> Communion with one's chosen deity comes from the
> study of sacred lore. (44)
> The perfection of pure contemplation comes from
> dedication to the Lord of Yoga. (45)

It should be recalled that three of the observances—ascetic practice, the study of sacred scripture, and dedication to the Lord of Yoga—receive emphasis at the opening of Part Two (2.1) as the components of the "active performance of yoga" (*kriyā-yoga*). Here, the specific benefits of these and the other observances are set forth.

The purification of the body makes one aware of its imperfections and the absurdity of attachment to it. This cultivation of aversion to the body also gives the yogi a distaste for physical contact with others and increases an inward focus.

Study involves intensive recitation of and meditation on sacred lore, especially the hymns or mantras of the ancient Vedas, which Hindus believe to possess the power to compel the attention of any deity invoked. Through the repetition of and meditation on specific mantras, the yogi can commune with a chosen deity, who can then aid his spiritual practice.

Dedication to the Lord characterizes the yogi's commitment to the discipline of the supreme yogi. The Lord—defined in Part One (1.24) as a distinct form of the spirit (*puruṣa*), who is unaffected by the forces of corruption or by actions and intentions—can serve as a model for the yogi to emulate.

POSTURE

> The posture of yoga is steady and easy. (46)
> It is realized by relaxing one's effort and resting like the cosmic serpent on the waters of infinity. (47)
> Then one is unconstrained by opposing dualities. (48)

Posture (*āsana*) is the relaxed positioning of the body that is necessary for practicing breath control and meditation. Patanjali compares it to resting like the cosmic serpent on the waters of infinity in the calm interval between cycles of universal creation and destruction. Ananta, "the infinite," is the cosmic serpent on whom the god Vishnu lies sleeping when the world dissolves at the end of each cosmic cycle, before the beginning of the next. Ananta may also refer to "the infinite" in a more abstract sense. This is the interpretation of the *Yogabhashya* commentary, which states that posture becomes perfect when effort to that end ceases, so that there is no more bodily movement, and when the mind is transformed into the infinite—that is, recognizes infinity as itself.

For Patanjali, the interior dimensions of yoga are impossible to attain unless one first pays attention to the body. Later traditions expand this aspect of yoga into a system of physically and spiritually efficacious postures, commonly known as *haṭha-yoga.*

Although Patanjali does not specify a particular posture, the lotus position has become, over time, the paradigm of all yogic postures. It is considered to be the perfect position for practicing breath control and meditation. Sitting with spine erect and one's legs folded into themselves, like the petals of a closed lotus, one can bring the entire body into a resting state. The relaxation that comes from sitting in the yogic posture fosters a state of equanimity, where pairs of opposites, such as heat and cold, pleasure and pain, self and other, cease to shape the yogi's awareness of existence.[13]

BREATH CONTROL

> When the posture of yoga is steady, then breath is controlled by regulation of the course of exhalation and inhalation. (49)

> The modification of breath in exhalation, inhalation, and retention is perceptible as deep and shallow breathing regulated by where the breath is held, for how long, and for how many cycles. (50)
> A fourth type of breath control goes beyond the range of exhalation and inhalation. (51)
> Then the cover over the light of truth dissolves. (52)
> And the mind is fit for concentration. (53)

Breath control (*prāṇāyāma*) involves the precise regulation of the rhythm of inhalation, retention, and exhalation of breath (*prāṇa*). The ability to control this vital force directs consciousness inward and concentrates it for meditation. In yoga, breath control is essential to further spiritual advancement. According to Patanjali, in order to control breathing one must focus on the place within the body where breath is held, adjust the length of time one inhales, retains, and exhales breath, and count the cycles of breathing.

Beyond the practice of disciplining normal breathing patterns, Patanjali suggests that there is a fourth mode of breathing, which transcends the three processes of exhalation, inhalation, and retention. This mode allows one to breathe effortlessly, thus dissipating the veil that obscures the true nature of things.[14] Although Patanjali gives no details, several commentators suggest that this process occurs when breathing virtually stops in pure contemplation (*samādhi*). Such minimal breathing is what allows advanced yogis to be buried alive for long periods without suffering ill effects.

WITHDRAWAL OF THE SENSES

When each sense organ severs contact with its objects, withdrawal of the senses corresponds to the intrinsic form of thought. (54)
From this comes complete control of the senses. (55)

Withdrawal (*pratyāhāra*) consists in isolating the senses from their objects. When the mind is made fit for concentration, the sense organs lose their attraction to their objects. The senses withdraw from external objects, allowing thought to turn inward. This in turn enables the yogi to practice the perfect discipline of the final three stages of yoga, which are delineated in Part Three. Withdrawal is thus the transitional phase in the process of introversion that culminates in concentration, meditation, and pure contemplation.

PART THREE

Perfect Discipline and Extraordinary Powers

PERFECT DISCIPLINE

Concentration is binding thought in one place. (1)

Meditation is focusing on a single conceptual flow. (2)

Pure contemplation is meditation that illumines the object alone, as if the subject were devoid of intrinsic form. (3)

Concentration, meditation, and pure contemplation focused on a single object constitute perfect discipline. (4)

The light of wisdom comes from mastery of perfect discipline. (5)

The practice of perfect discipline is achieved in stages. (6)

In contrast with the prior limbs of yoga, the final triad is internal. (7)

Yet it is only an external limb of seedless contemplation. (8)

This section defines the final three limbs of the eightfold way, collectively the hyperconscious state known as "perfect discipline" (*saṃyama*). Concentration, meditation, and pure contemplation are the internal limbs of yoga, which concentrate the yogi's energy and free his thought of constraints, allowing it to experience limitless knowledge and powers, such as the ability to know past and future, enter into other bodies, and understand the languages of animals and birds.

Each of the three limbs of perfect discipline is a stage in the process of achieving spiritual freedom. Concentration (*dhāraṇā*) involves focusing attention on a particular spot, such as the navel, the heart, the tip of the nose, or an internally visualized image. Meditation (*dhyāna*) is unwavering attention to a single object—a continuous flow of attention that, like the flow of oil, is uninterrupted by any extraneous idea. Pure contemplation (*samādhi*) is achieved when the meditative subject is so absorbed in the object of meditation that the distinction between subject and object disappears. The observer, transcending all awareness of a separate personal identity, takes the form of the object contemplated, attains complete control over it, and is absorbed in it—obliterating the artificial, conceptual separation between the observer and object.

Patanjali closes his account of the limbs of perfect discipline by reminding us that even pure contemplation (*samādhi*) is not the deepest level in the process of spiritual transformation. Beyond it, at the culmination of yogic practice, is seedless contemplation (*nirbīja-samādhi*), which was defined at the close of Part One (1.47). Seedless contemplation—the absolute freedom that exists when all thought has ceased—will be the subject of the fourth and final section of the text.

THE TRANSFORMATIONS OF THOUGHT AND MATERIAL NATURE

The transformation of thought leading toward its own cessation is accompanied by moments of cessation, when subliminal impressions of mental distraction are overcome and those of cessation emerge in their place. (9)

From subliminal impressions of these moments, the flow of tranquility is constant. (10)

The transformation of thought toward pure contemplation occurs when concern for all external objects declines and psychic focus arises. (11)

The transformation of thought toward psychic focus occurs when a concept is equally at rest or arising. (12)

By extension, these transformations of thought explain the transformations of nature's properties, characteristics, and conditions, which occur in material elements and sense organs. (13)

The substratum underlying the essential properties of material nature endures whether these properties are at rest, arising, or unmanifest. (14)

Variation in the sequence of properties causes differences in the transformations of nature. (15)

This set of aphorisms is dense with technical specifications. The phenomenon under examination here is the imperceptible sequence of transformations that leads to the cessation of thought. Patanjali begins by describing the first, momentary experiences of meditative calm that become the basis for achieving an absolute calm. These transformations are possible because all thought is shaped by subliminal impressions (*saṃskāra*), which are left in the mind after any experience and which shape new thoughts. As explained, these subliminal impressions are of two kinds, one detrimental to spiritual development, the other beneficial. One kind distracts thought and makes it restless; the other calms thought and brings it to rest.

When attention wavers, subliminal impressions of distraction come to the fore to obstruct the process of meditation. These can be suppressed by evoking a subliminal impression of cessation through a form of "passive" meditation; otherwise, the impression of cessation is merely another distraction. Patanjali seems to be saying that at the very moment thought arises there can be an instantaneous cessation of thought that produces a waveless, unagitated flow of subliminal impressions. These impressions suffuse thought with a calm that is conducive to perfect discipline (*saṃyama*). In this process, thought about a wide range of objects contracts into a point of focus on a single object. When thought is completely focused on a single point, calm and active thought merge and one achieves a state of pure contemplation.[15]

Patanjali extends his analysis of the transformations of thought to explain transformations in the elements and senses, which are characterized as changes in the properties, characteristics, and conditions of any object. The commentators discuss the technical meaning of aphorism 3.13 at great length, illustrating the discussion with the example of the changes undergone by a clay pot. The natural progression of creation involves a sequential order—clay as dust, the lump of clay, the clay pot, the shards of the broken pot. The point is that through all of its transformations the clay material never loses its essential nature (cf. 4.14). The analogy between the transformations of thought and the transformations of objects in the material world enables the yogi, who has experienced these changes, to understand the universal cycle of creation and destruction. This gives him knowledge of the past and future.

THE POWERS OF EXTRAORDINARY KNOWLEDGE

> Knowledge of the past and future comes from perfect discipline of the three transformations of thought. (16)
> Confusion arises from erroneously identifying words, objects, and ideas with one another; knowledge of the cries of all creatures comes through perfect discipline of the distinctions between them. (17)
> Through direct perception of one's subliminal impressions, one has knowledge of former births. (18)
> Through direct perception of the cognitive process, one has knowledge of the thoughts of others. (19)
> But this does not involve knowledge of the underlying object of thought since that is not one's object of perception. (20)

The perfect discipline (*saṃyama*) of the three transformations of thought refers again to the integration of concentration, meditation, and pure contemplation. This leads to extraordinary forms of knowledge and power. All of the powers Patanjali will go on to discuss manifest themselves to the yogi in the hyperconsciousness of perfect discipline. Just as the inner eye of an adept in meditation can bring a visual image to life, so the meditative consciousness can actualize powers that are unimaginable at conventional levels of thought. What we experience in dreams can also take on a vivid physical reality.

Perhaps the most direct analogy for the operation of the powers is the idea of what theoretical physicists call "thought experiments" (*gedanken experimenten*), in contrast to physical experiments. We accept without question the ability of Albert Einstein to perform his famous thought experiment of an elevator falling through space, or the ability of contemporary theorists of relativity like Stephen Hawking to talk about a world of more than twenty dimensions.[16] In each case the thought experiment requires a relaxation of conventional conceptual constraints, freeing the scientist to grasp extraordinary possibilities that may explain physical phenomena in profoundly new ways.

Patanjali's account of the specific powers is terse, leaving their exact meaning ambiguous in some cases, but the general nature of these powers emerges from the examples. The power to know the thought of others develops from the yogi's highly developed sensitivity to the limitless possibilities of the cognitive process. Patanjali says that the yogi perceives what the other person is thinking without knowing the actual object prompting that idea. This occurs because the object of the yogi's knowledge is the other person's conception, not what he or she is actually perceiving. As the commentators explain: if the yogi reads another person's mind when that mind is perceiving a rope as a snake, he sees the idea of a snake; he does not see the rope that is giving rise to the other person's perception.

FURTHER POWERS OF PERFECT DISCIPLINE

From perfect discipline of the body's form, one can become invisible by paralyzing the power to perceive one's body and blocking the contact of light from one's eyes. (21)

From perfect discipline of the immediate and remote effects of action, or from omens, one has foreknowledge of death. (22)

From perfect discipline of friendship, compassion, joy, and impartiality, one has their strengths. (23)

From perfect discipline of the strength of an animal such as an elephant, one gains that strength. (24)

From placing light on the mind's activity, one has knowledge of that which is subtle, hidden, and distant. (25)

From perfect discipline of the sun, one has knowledge of the worlds. (26)

From perfect discipline of the moon, one has knowledge of the arrangement of the stars. (27)

From perfect discipline of the polestar, one has knowledge of the movement of the stars. (28)

From perfect discipline of the circle of the navel, one has knowledge of the body's arrangement. (29)

From perfect discipline of the cavity in the throat, hunger and thirst are subdued. (30)

From perfect discipline of the "tortoise vein," one's being becomes steady. (31)

From perfect discipline of the light in the head, one gets a vision of the perfected beings. (32)
From intuition, one knows everything. (33)
From perfect discipline of the heart, one has full consciousness of one's thought. (34)

The concentrated energy that accumulates through the perfect discipline of concentration, meditation, and pure contemplation extends the practitioner's powers, thereby enabling the laws of nature to be defied. The yogi develops extraordinary states of consciousness and physical capacities such as invisibility, superhuman strength, knowledge of past and future lives, knowledge of the workings of the cosmos and the microcosm of the body, as well as control over the physical needs of hunger and thirst.

Among the disciplines, control of the "tortoise vein" is somewhat obscure; according to ancient Indian anatomy, the tortoise vein is one of the vessels that run through the body. Vyasa identifies it as having the shape of a tortoise and being located in the chest. The suggestion here is that perfect discipline of this vessel makes one like a tortoise—steady, capable of withdrawing into a hard shell and immobilizing the senses.

The "light in the head" probably refers to the inner, or third, eye, which gives one insight into the ways of perfected beings, or *siddha*s, the adepts of Hindu, Buddhist, and Jain spiritual practice, who have transcended the constraints of the phenomenal world. Perfect discipline of one's intuition and heart generates omniscience and total self-consciousness. In Patanjali's view, it is through meditation on the heart that one becomes conscious of one's inner being, which is preliminary to gaining knowledge of the spirit (*puruṣa*).

KNOWLEDGE OF THE SPIRIT

> Worldly experience is caused by a failure to differentiate between the lucid quality of nature and the spirit. From perfect discipline of the distinction between spirit as the subject of itself and the lucid quality of nature as a dependent object, one gains knowledge of the spirit. (35)
>
> This knowledge engenders intuitive forms of hearing, touch, sight, taste, and smell. (36)
>
> If they become a distraction these powers of perfection are impediments to pure contemplation. (37)

Even for an advanced practitioner of yoga, involvement in the phenomenal world continues as long as one fails to discriminate between spirit (*puruṣa*) and the lucid quality of nature (*sattva-guṇa*), the most perfect aspect of the material world. Being material, nature's lucidity is mutable, whereas the spirit is immutable. The spirit does not perceive a knowable object in the conventional way. Rather, it is "pure consciousness": when the yogi concentrates on the distinction between spirit and nature's lucidity, he has knowledge of the spirit. The spirit is not known by the idea of spirit, since ideas belong to the realm of conceptual thought. It is the spirit alone that knows itself.

The yogi's aim is not to reach the apex of the material condition, however pure, but to realize his innermost spiritual being. By confusing the perfection of the material world with the spirit, desire for worldly perfection interferes with spiritual attainment.

The relation between knowledge and power is direct, but Patanjali cautions that the powers that knowledge manifests can fool one into overlooking the goal, which is seedless contemplation and total freedom from the material world. The powers are only representations of spiritual development, weak analogies for the ultimate supermundane goal of freedom. This idea is elaborated in aphorisms 3.50–51.

MASTERY OF THE PHYSICAL WORLD

From loosening the fetters of bondage to the body and
from awareness of the body's fluidity, one's thought can
enter into the body of another. (38)
From mastery of the vital breath rising in the body, one
does not sink into water, mud, or thorns, but rather rises
above them. (39)
From mastery of the breath of fire in the belly, one
acquires a fiery radiance. (40)
From perfect discipline of the relation between the ear
and space, one has divine hearing. (41)
From perfect discipline of the relation between the body
and space and from contemplative poise in which the
body is as light as cotton, one can move through
space. (42)
The turning of thought without reference to the
external world is called "the great disembodied
thought"; from this the veil that obscures the light is
destroyed. (43)

> From perfect discipline of the gross, intrinsic, subtle, relational, and purposive aspects of the elements of matter, one attains mastery over them. (44)
> Then extraordinary powers appear, such as the power to be as small as an atom, as well as bodily perfection and immunity from the constraints of matter. (45)

The physical powers described here all depend on mastery over subtle aspects of the body and its relation to other dimensions of the material world, such as thought and space. When one is able to free thought from egoistical attachment to one's own body, thought is able to penetrate other bodies and inhabit them mentally.

Breath control as one of the main limbs of yogic practice has been outlined in the previous section. Here, mastery over specific aspects of the breathing process is said to confer special powers. There are five vital breaths (*prāṇa*) in the Yoga system. Among these the rising breath (*udāna*) functions from the tip of the nose to the head. Mastery of it gives one the ability to walk over things that would ordinarily be impediments, such as water, mud, or thorns. The digestive breath (*samāna*) has its seat in the stomach and intestines, and its fiery quality is essential to digestion. Its mastery gives the body the glowing aura of fire.

The notion that the entire physical world, including the body, is composed of five material elements (*bhūta*) is found throughout ancient Indian philosophy. The five elements are earth, water, fire, air, and ether or space. In Patanjali's view, perfect discipline of the five elements in all their aspects endows the yogi with eight supernatural powers. These include becoming tiny or gigantic, light or heavy, capable of attaining anything, irresistible, omnipotent, and dominant over the creation and destruction of the elements.[17] These powers make the yogi's body perfect and immune to the natural forces of corruption, like aging and death. Because he is beyond constraint by the elements of matter, the solidity of earth does not restrict the action of his body, so that it can penetrate dense substances like rock. Water does not wet it; fire cannot burn it; the wind cannot move it.

OTHER POWERS

> Bodily perfection includes beauty, grace, strength, and a diamond's hard glow. (46)
>
> From perfect discipline of the receptive, intrinsic, egoistic, relational, and purposive functions of the sense organs, one attains mastery over them. (47)
>
> From this one acquires quickness of mind, perception without the aid of the senses, and mastery over primordial matter. (48)
>
> For one who is attentive to the distinction between the lucid perfection of nature and the spirit, omniscience and power over all states of existence result. (49)

Just as perfect discipline of the five elements in all their aspects gives the yogi powers drawn from them (3.44), so perfect discipline of the various functions of the sense organs bestows mastery over the causes, processes, and objects of sensation. According to highly technical ancient Indian theories of sense perception, to which Patanjali is alluding here, each of the sense organs has five functions. If one takes sound as an example, the general idea is that a sound excites the organ of hearing, which activates an individualistic perception of the sound, which causes knowledge of the sound.[18] When the senses are mastered, they can in turn be transcended, giving one immediate apprehension of all the dimensions of nature.

Omniscience and mastery over all of existence depend on being able to discriminate between the lucid aspect of material nature (*sattva-guṇa*) and the spirit (*puruṣa*), an idea introduced above (3.35). The yogi who knows all of nature in its subtlest perfection knows all there is to know in the world of existence; such a yogi also knows that this world is essentially distinct from the spirit.

THE LIMITATIONS OF THE POWERS

From dispassion even toward these powers, freedom of
the spirit occurs with the destruction of the seeds of
sin. (50)
One should avoid enthusiasm or pride in the
enticements of the gods, lest harmful attachments
recur. (51)
From perfect discipline of moments and their sequence
in time, one has the knowledge born of
discrimination. (52)
Through discrimination one comprehends differences
of origin, characteristic, or position that distinguish two
seemingly similar things. (53)

> Knowledge born of discrimination is transcendent, comprehensive, concerned with all states of things, and instantaneous. (54)
>
> Absolute freedom occurs when the lucidity of material nature and spirit are in pure equilibrium. (55)

In order to achieve absolute freedom from nature, the yogi must transcend the limitations on the spirit that even knowledge and extraordinary powers impose. Here, the practitioner is warned that the powers gained through perfect discipline might lead the unwary astray by inspiring pride, egoism, and new cravings. In order to realize freedom, the yogi must cultivate dispassion toward the extraordinary insights and capabilities that his discipline has revealed, and hone his discriminative powers to penetrate deeper levels of reality.

Mastery of time in its minute components and in its order enables the yogi to notice the most subtle differences between similar things, which people of lesser knowledge see as equal. It confers on him the ultimate power to distinguish between the perfection of nature and spirit. But even this distinction, crucial in the psychological process, is irrelevant when the true equilibrium of spirit and matter is restored.

PART FOUR

Absolute Freedom

TRANSFORMATIONS OF REBIRTH

The powers of perfection that arise through pure
contemplation may also accrue from magical herbs,
spells, or ascetic practice in a previous birth. (1)
The transformation from one species into another at
birth results from an overflow of material forces. (2)
There is no efficient cause of these material forces, but a
breaching of the barriers that contain them, as when a
farmer irrigates fields. (3)

In this final section of the *Yoga Sutra,* the aphorisms are structured to reiterate and reinforce analyses of the relation between the observing spirit and the material world that have been presented in other parts of the text. An understanding of the causal network of action, thought, memory, and subliminal impressions is crucial to developing the discrimination that liberates spirit from the corrupting forces of the material world.

This section is quite elliptical in places because Patanjali assumes that the reader already has a grasp of the basic concepts of his analysis, as well as some technical Sankhya ideas on causality. Various ideas about change and causality are introduced to prepare the ground for a deeper insight into the relation between thought (*citta*) and action (*karma*). Fundamental to Patanjali's view is the more general Indian theory that thought and action are involved in an endless round of reciprocal causality that repeats itself through many cycles of rebirth. Actions create memory traces, which are stored in memory and fuel the mental processes. The store of subliminal impressions is obliterated only when the chain of causal relations is broken, liberating the spirit from its attachment to the world of physical and mental activity.

According to Sankhya-Yoga cosmology, material nature is like energy in potential form, always ready to flow out and actualize itself if the barriers are removed, like the flow of water in an irrigation system controlled by sluices. The notion of a reservoir of material forces, built up through natural evolution and experience, explains how the same body has different forms in childhood, youth, and old age, or how a seed changes into a fig tree.

Patanjali begins this section by shifting his perspective on the powers of perfection. Having explained them in Part Three as the result of perfect discipline, which culminates in pure contemplation (*samādhi*), he now presents the notion that the powers can be acquired through other means, which carry over from one birth to the next. This is a prelude to a restatement of some basic ideas introduced in Part Three (beginning at 3.9) about how thought, action, and material nature undergo transformations.

THE TRANSFORMATION OF THOUGHT

> Individual thoughts are constructed from a measure of egoism. (4)
> A single thought produces the diverse activities of many thoughts. (5)
> A thought born of meditation leaves no trace of subliminal intention. (6)

Here Patanjali sets up a contrast between thought that arises from egoism (*asmitā,* one of the afflictions) and thought that arises from meditation (2.3). Egoism, in which everything is considered in relation to oneself, derives from the false identification of spirit with matter. Egoistic thoughts each cause multiple other thoughts in turn. By contrast, a thought that arises from meditation does not give rise to further thoughts or to subliminal intention (*āśava*), memories of past experience that lie dormant, later to impel an individual to action.[19]

THE TRANSFORMATION OF ACTION

> The action of a yogi is neither black nor white; that of others is black or white, or black and white. (7)
> Each color of action leaves memory traces corresponding to the fruition of the action. (8)
> From the uniformity of memory and subliminal impressions, the continuity of subliminal impressions is sustained, even through interruptions of birth, place, and time. (9)

> These subliminal impressions are without beginning because the desires that sustain them are eternal. (10)
> Since the subliminal impressions are held together by the interdependence of cause and effect, when these cease to exist, the impressions also cease to exist. (11)

The nature of action (*karma*) is analogous to the nature of thought. The classification as black, white, black and white, and neither black nor white is one of the many ways that the repercussions of action are described. Black marks the action of evil; white represents religious activities that are independent of external means and cause no harm; action that is black and white lies in between. The action of a yogi is neither black nor white, because his store of *karma* has been exhausted through renunciation of the fruits of action, and he harbors no belief that "I am the doer."

In Patanjali's view, actions produce effects only if one feels attachment to them, thereby creating memory traces. The store of these subliminal impressions is obliterated only when the chain of causal relations is broken—when there is neither doer, nor act of doing, nor object.

THE REALITY OF MATERIAL THINGS AND THE STRUCTURE OF THOUGHT

> Past and future time exist within all things because the properties of nature move at different tempos. (12)
> These properties of nature, whether visible or subtle, are the essence of material things. (13)

A thing has reality because it remains unique
throughout various transformations. (14)
Although an object remains constant, people's
perceptions of it differ because they associate different
thoughts with it. (15)
If an object is not structured within a coherent thought,
will it still exist, even though unknown? (16)
A thing is known or not known to thought depending
on whether thought is colored by it. (17)

The issue here is whether or not the reality of an object is dependent on the uniform structure of thought, which is itself part of material nature. For Patanjali, the reality of a thing is consistent and independent of subjective thought, but the mutability of thought makes the object appear to change. An object is known only when it arises in thought. Underlying this argument is the basic presupposition that material nature is real; what is illusory is the false identification thought makes between material nature and spirit.

In its turnings, thought may or may not recognize an object, but this does not negate the object's reality. In earlier sutras Patanjali also asserts the reality of external things, with an implied contrast to idealist views.[20] For him, discriminative knowledge is not possible without a full understanding of the process of how knowledge of the world is acquired and the relation of this thought process to the spirit.

These ideas are at least in part based on a debate among Buddhist scholars of the time.[21] According to the commentators, these aphorisms are addressed to Buddhist idealists who are deceived by the resemblance of thought and the spirit. These philosophers hold that all objects are mental constructs, that there is no objective reality, and that nothing exists in the absence of a knowing subject. In Patanjali's epistemology, the independent existence of the objective world does not engender a uniform perception of objects but rather produces different responses in different subjects.

THOUGHT AND SPIRIT

> The spirit, never subject to change, is master of the turnings of thought, which it always knows. (18)
> Since thought is an object of perception, it cannot illuminate itself. (19)
> Nor can both thought and its object be comprehended simultaneously. (20)
> If a thought is the object of another thought, there is an infinite regression from intelligence to intelligence, and a confusion of memory. (21)
> Awareness of its own intelligence occurs when thought assumes the form of the spirit through consciousness that leaves no trace. (22)

Patanjali now expands on the relationship between thought and spirit. Since thought belongs to the phenomenal world, it is a knowable object. Unlike the spirit, which is self-luminous, thought cannot know itself. Thought is dependent on the reflected light of the spirit for knowledge of its own processes, just as the moon depends on the light of the sun. If thought were self-luminous, it would be able to conceive of itself and its objects at the same time, but it cannot.

If the thought process were the object of another thought process, which was in turn the object of another, there would be an infinite regression. There would thus be endless turnings of thought, producing an endless store of unordered memory, which would create troublesome impressions (cf. 2.17).

This section again stresses that the way the spirit knows is distinct from ordinary thought. It is the spirit's illumination of thought that enables thought to understand its own structures and component parts. Thought can only penetrate intelligence (*buddhi*), which is one of its components, when it operates without dependence on the restless turnings of thought. This special kind of understanding (*citi*) leaves no impression and does not reflect back on itself. Instead, it produces a self-awareness that liberates thought from its inherent limits.

THOUGHT AND THE OBSERVER

> Colored by both the observer and the phenomenal world, thought can take everything as its object. (23)
>
> Variegated by countless traces of memory, thought works by making associations, for the sake of a purpose beyond itself. (24)
>
> One who sees the distinction between the lucid quality of nature and the observer ceases to cultivate a personal reality. (25)
>
> Then, deep in discrimination, thought gravitates toward freedom. (26)

Patanjali once more appears to be countering the Buddhist idealists, who hold that nothing exists in the absence of a knowing subject. By contrast, Patanjali's belief in the independent existence of the world means that an object may be known or not known. An object is known only if thought is colored by that object—so thought may or may not know an object, which makes thought unstable. Spirit, in contrast, is stable and unchanging. Thought's special character resides in its capacity to intuit even what is beyond thought, including the spirit, for whose sake the thought process works (cf. 2.17–27).

Patanjali seems to be pointing to the fact that thought operates through association, structuring the disparate objects of experience and subliminal impressions into categories for knowing. Thus thought cannot be self-directed but must instead exist for the sake of something else—namely, the observing spirit, which, unlike thought, does not depend on associations in order to know.

When the yogi's thought is cultivated to the degree that it can discriminate between the purest aspect of the material world and the observing spirit, any egoistic sense of personal identity ceases (cf. 4.4). Then thought can terminate in yogic calm.

THE CESSATION OF ACTIONS AND FORCES OF CORRUPTION

When there are lapses in discrimination, distracting
concepts arise from the store of subliminal
impressions. (27)

> Like the forces of corruption, these ideas can be eliminated by reversing their course and by meditation. (28)
>
> For one who seeks no gain even in vast knowledge, perpetual discrimination is called "the essential cloud of pure contemplation." (29)
>
> On account of this, forces of corruption and actions cease to exist. (30)

The ideas presented here recapitulate what Patanjali introduced earlier (see 2.10–12). The pure contemplation called "the essential-cloud-contemplation" (*dharma-megha-samādhi*) is a state in which pure contemplation pours knowledge to keep thought discriminative, calm, and effortless, just as a cloud pours rain. Given the complexity of the term *dharma,* this phrase has been interpreted in varied ways by commentators, but its most basic meaning seems to construe best with the sense of the aphorisms in this section.[22]

THE KNOWLEDGE THAT ENDS IN FREEDOM

> Then the infinity of knowledge, released from impurities that obscure everything, leaves little to be known. (31)
>
> This infinite knowledge means an end to the sequence of transformations in material things, their purpose now fulfilled. (32)

> Sequence corresponds to a series of moments
> perceivable at the end of a process of
> transformation. (33)
> Freedom is a reversal of the evolutionary course of
> material things, which are empty of meaning for the
> spirit; it is also the power of consciousness in a state of
> true identity. (34)

In these final aphorisms, the text concludes by spiraling back on itself. Patanjali began the *Yoga Sutra* by defining yoga in terms of the true identity of the observing spirit, which is realized through total cessation of the turnings of thought. He ends by stating that the knowledge acquired through the practice of yoga becomes infinite knowledge. It is an omniscience that allows the observer to become independent from the temporal constraints of the changing world of nature.

Thought is bound in time; thinking about the world depends on a temporal sequence of ideas. Since infinite knowledge knows everything in the present, the evolutionary process that gives nature its structure and meaning ceases to be relevant. The workings of nature are empty of meaning for the spirit (*puruṣārtha-śūnya*) that is liberated. In a real sense, Patanjali has established what it means in terms of yoga for one's spirit to achieve its true identity as observer to the world—a witness rather than a suffering participant in a world of ceaseless, volatile change.

REFERENCE MATTER

A NOTE ON TRANSLITERATION

A dual system of transliteration has been adopted in the present work. So that the main body of the text may remain accessible to a broad range of readers, proper names appear there without diacritics (thus Patanjali and *Yoga Sutra*). For the benefit of readers who do have some knowledge of Sanskrit, however, diacritics have been retained whenever technical terms appear within parentheses, as well as on all names and terms in the reference matter (thus Patañjali and *Yoga Sūtra*). For interested readers, the following guide to the pronunciation of Sanskrit words may also prove useful.

a	like the *u* in h*u*t
ā	like the *a* in f*a*ther
i	like the *i* in k*i*n
ī	like the *ee* in k*ee*p
u	like the *u* in p*u*t
ū	like the *oo* in h*oo*t
ṛ	like the *ri* in *ri*ff
ṝ	like the *ree* in *ree*l
e	like the *ay* in pl*ay*
ai	like the *i* in sm*i*le
o	like the *o* in h*o*me
au	like the *ow* in g*ow*n

Syllables that contain long vowels (*ā, ī, ū, ṝ*) or dipthongs (*e, o, ai, au*) receive stress. An *ṃ* has the effect of nasalizing the preceding vowel but may be approximated by an English *m*. The *ḥ* is a rough breathing, which causes the preceding vowel to echo.

For the most part, consonants are pronounced as in English. A *g* is always hard, as in *g*o; the *ch* and *c* are both *ch* sounds (as in *ch*in). An *ṅ* is pronounced like the *ng* in su*ng;* a *ñ* is a *ny* sound, just like the Spanish *ñ*. Both *ś* and *ṣ* sound much like the English *sh* (*sh*ip), whereas an *s* without a diacritic is just *s* (as in *s*un).

Unlike English, Sanskrit distinguishes between unaspirated and aspirated consonants; the latter are written with a following *h* (*kh, gh, ch, jh, th, dh, ṭh, ḍh, ph, bh*). To speakers of English, though, they sound essentially the same as their unaspirated equivalents. (The difference is that between the sound of the *k* in s*k*in—which is unaspirated—and *k*in.) Thus, for example, *t* and *th* are both pronounced much like the *t* in hi*t*. The consonants *ṭ, ṭh, ḍ, ḍh, ṇ,* and *ṣ* are retroflex, pronounced similarly to their nonretroflex counterparts but with the tongue further back, touching the roof of the mouth.

KEYWORDS IN THE *YOGA SUTRA*

Many words in the text have technical meanings that are replete with complex histories and relations to other philosophical traditions—Hindu, Buddhist, and Jain. As commentators have pointed out, Patañjali is often carrying on an internal dialogue with alternate views on specific points. It is not my intention to present this level of textual criticism. Readers who wish to explore Patañjali's technical vocabulary more deeply are referred to the following works:

Aranya, Hariharananda. *Yoga Philosophy of Patanjali,* with Vyāsa's commentary, translated by P. N. Mukherji. Albany: SUNY Press, 1983.

Dasgupta, Surendranath: *A Study of Patanjali.* Calcutta: Calcutta University, 1920; 2d ed. Delhi: Motilal Banarsidass, 1989.

Eliade, Mircea. *Yoga: Immortality and Freedom,* 2d ed. Princeton: Princeton University Press, 1969.

Feuerstein, Georg. *The Philosophy of Classical Yoga.* Manchester: Manchester University Press, 1980.

———. *The Yoga-Sūtra of Patanjali.* Rochester, Vt.: Inner Traditions, 1989.

Woods, James Haughton. *The Yoga-System of Patañjali,* Harvard Oriental Series, vol. 17. Cambridge, Mass.: Harvard University Press, 1914; repr. Delhi: Motilal Banarsidass, 1966. Includes translations of the commentaries of Vyāsa and Vācaspati Miśra.

The following glossary provides basic definitions of Patañjali's core vocabulary to which the reader can refer whenever these terms occur in the text. In the *Yoga Sūtra* Patañjali frequently draws on ancient philosophical terms and redefines them within the text itself. In order to reflect the technical style of the Sanskrit original, I have tried to use specific English equivalents of Patañjali's keywords consistently throughout the translation.

ACTION (*karma*) 1.24; 2.12; 3.22; 4.7, 30; any action, but particularly action that has repercussions in this or the next life.

ASCETIC PRACTICE (*tapas*) 2.1, 32, 43; 4.1; this word literally means "heat," that is, the hot energy that is generated in the body by means of hardships and privations (fasting, sleeping on the bare ground, wandering in the wild, exposure to heat and cold, etc.).

AWARENESS (*saṃvedana*) 3.38; 4.22; cf. feeling (*vedana*) 3.36; these terms denote especially the act of perceiving as a result of sensation.

BASIS, FOUNDATION (*pratiṣṭhā*) 1.8; 2.35, 36, 37, 38; 4.34; the basic status or form of something. In Part Two, the term denotes a state of steadfast perseverance.

BIRTH (*jāti*) 2.13, 31; 3.18, 53 ("origin"); 4.2, 9; the condition of entering a new body, which is caused by previous actions and leads to the accumulation of new karmic residues. Birth may be in a high or low status.

BREATH (*prāṇa*) 1.34; breath control (*prāṇāyāma*) 2.29; life is sustained by the movement of various types of breath in the body. Breath control is meant to regulate these breaths strictly, and even to bring them to a halt.

CAUSE (*hetu*) 2.17, 23, 24; 3.15; 4.11; causation, state of being a cause (*hetutva*) 2.14.

CELIBACY (*brahmacarya*) 2.30, 38; one of the five moral principles, *brahmacarya* is abstinence from sexual activity and the retention of semen, which contains vital power.

CESSATION, CESSATION OF THE TURNINGS OF THOUGHT (*nirodha*) 1.2, 12, 51; 3.9; this is both a means and an absolute goal. As a means, the word denotes the momentary poise experienced when all thought ceases during the final stages of yogic practice. Cf. the Buddhist notion of cessation, as in the doctrine of the Four Noble Truths.

CONCENTRATION (*dhāraṇā*) 2.29, 53; 3.1; (*avadhāraṇa*) 4.20; the focusing of attention on a particular spot, such as the navel, the heart, the tip of the nose, or any external object.

CONCEPT (*pratyaya*), namely, the concept by which a thing is known; the word is often difficult to translate, especially where it is used in a less technical sense (as in Part One) 1.10, 18, 19; 2.20; 3.2, 12, 17, 19, 35; 4.27. On *abhāva-pratyaya* (1.10) and *bhava-pratyaya* (1.19), see the commentary.

CONCEPTUALIZATION (*vikalpa*) 1.6, 9, 42; one of the five "turnings of thought" (*citta-vṛtti*), *vikalpa* is the tendency of thought to construct a reality that has no basis beyond individual subjectivity, involving a confusion of words, objects designated by words, and meaning. Frequently translated as fancy, *vikalpa* rather refers to a conceptualization of the world based on verbal knowledge. An important term in the vocabulary of Buddhist philosophy as well.

CONDITION (*avasthā*) 3.13; (*avasthāna*) 1.3; the changing condition of the spirit that is restored to its pure state through yoga (1.3).

CONJECTURE (*vitarka*) 1.17; 2.33, 34; (*savitarka*) 1.42; (*nirvitarka*) 1.43; thinking based on gross evidence, in contrast with *vicāra,* which refers to fine-grained reasoning; conjectural thought that may give one perverse ideas.

CONSCIOUSNESS (*citi*) 4.22, 34; spirit's direct apprehension of itself.

CONSEQUENCES, MATURING OF THE FRUIT OF ACTION, FRUITION OF ACTION (*vipāka*) 1.24; 2.13; 4.8; literally, the "ripening" of the fruits of action, which has its origin in the "seeds" of thought; cf. seed (*bīja*) and fruit (*phala*).

CONTEMPLATION, PURE CONTEMPLATION (*samādhi*) 1.20, 46, 51; 2.2, 29, 45; 3.3, 11, 37; 4.1, 29; the final stage of yogic practice. This term, resistant to simple translation, has been rendered by such words as "trance." It is an integrated state of complete concentration, meditation, and pure contemplation in which the spirit is aware of its fundamental isolation from material nature and its own absolute integrity. This state is achieved when the meditating subject is absorbed in the object of meditation so that the distinction between subject and object disappears. Patañjali's clearest definition of *samādhi* is "meditation that illumines the object alone, as if the subject were devoid of its own identity" (3.3). There are two levels of contemplation, which Patañjali calls "seeded" (*sabīja*) and "seedless" (*nirbīja*), the former being transitive and limited by consciousness, the latter being intransitive and superconscious. Seedless contemplation is also called "essential-cloud" (*dharma-megha*) contemplation (4.29), in which the yogi becomes indifferent even to omniscience and omnipotence. Parallel to this is the Buddhist term *dharma-megha,* which refers to the final stage of the bodhisattva's path to perfection. Cf. perfect discipline (*saṃyama*).

CONTEMPLATIVE POISE (*samāpatti*) 1.41, 42; 2.47; 3.42; mental absorption in which thought becomes one with the object of thought. In contemplative poise thought is like a flawless crystal, assuming the form of the object meditated on. *Samāpatti* is closely related to *sabīja-samādhi,* for the attainment of which it is essential.

CONTROL (*vaśīkāra*) 1.15, 40; (*vaśyatā*) 2.55; mastery over one's own senses and their cravings, which leads to mastery over external things (1.40).

CORRUPTION, FORCE OF CORRUPTION (*kleśa*) 1.24; 2.2, 3; 3.12; 4.28, 30; *kliṣṭa-akliṣṭa,* "corrupted or immune to the forces of corruption," 1.5. The five forces of corruption—ignorance, egoism, passion, hatred, and clinging to life—are forces that motivate action in the phenomenal world. They bear comparison with the *kleśa*s of Buddhist philosophy, corruptive forces that include passion, hatred, and ignorance or delusion. In the Tantric Buddhist Wheel of Life, they are represented by three creatures at the hub of phenomenal existence: the cock, the snake, and the pig.

DISCERNMENT, THE ABILITY TO DISCRIMINATE BETWEEN DIFFERENT OBJECTS (*khyāti*) 1.16; 2.5; 3.49; focused discrimination (*viveka-khyāti*) 2.26, 28; 4.29.

DISCIPLINE (*yoga*) 1.1, 2; 2.1, 28; the discipline for achieving spiritual freedom; cf. the practicer of yoga (*yogin*) 4.7; aptitude, fitness (*yogyatā*) 2.53; (*yogyatva*) 2.41; correspondence (*pratiyogin*) 4.33; effecting, producing (*prayojaka*) 4.5; (*aprayojaka*) 4.3; connection (*saṃyoga*) 2.17, 23, 25; communion (*samprayoga*) 2.44; use, application (*viniyoga*) 3.6. See also perfect discipline (*saṃyama*).

DISCRIMINATION (*viveka*) 2.26, 28; 3. 52, 54; 4.26, 29; *vivekin* 2.15; the ability to discriminate between the self and what is not self (e.g., between the spiritual and the material).

DISPASSION (*vairāgya*) 1.12, 15; 3.50; defined by Patañjali as "the sign of mastery over the craving for sensuous objects." This probably refers, as the commentators suggest, to the objectives of ancient Vedic sacred lore and sacrifice, which are long life, material rewards, and ultimately heaven; cf. absence of craving (*vitṛṣṇa*) 1.15; (*vaitṛṣṇya*) 1.16.

DISTINCTION (*bheda*) 4.3, 5, 12, 15; breach, break.

EGOISM (*asmitā*) 1.17; 2.3, 6; 3.47; 4.4; one of the afflictions (2.3), *asmitā* is the egocentric attitude in which everything is considered in relation to oneself. In Patañjali's system, it derives from the false identification of spirit with matter, of the observer with the phenomenal world. In Sāṃkhya, the parallel concept is the "egomaker" (*ahaṃkāra*), which is an evolute of matter.

ELEMENT (*bhūta*) 2.18; 3.13, 44; referring to one or all of the five material elements: earth, water, fire, air, and ether or space; creature 3.17; cf. 3.20.

ERROR (*viparyaya*) 1.6, 8; false knowledge, which has no basis in fact.

ESSENCE, ESSENTIAL BEING, SELF (*ātman*) 2.5, 21, 41; 4.13; the existence of a self (*ātmabhāva*) 4.25; absence of self (*anātman*) 2.5; essential (*ātmaka*) 2.18; inner, interior (*adhyātma*) 1.47; this term designates the inner, unchanging, immaterial essence of a person.

EXISTENCE (*bhāva*) 3.48, 49; 4.25; nonexistence, absence (*abhāva*) 1.10, 29; 2.25; 4.11; "becoming," i.e., the phenomenal world (*bhāva*) 1.19; bringing about (*bhāvana*) 1.28; 2.33, 34; cultivation, fostering (*bhāvanā*) 1.33; 2.2; 4.25; emergence (*prādurbhāva*) 3.9, 45.

EXPERIENCE (*bhoga*) 2.13, 18; 3.35; the experience of pleasure and pain involved in acting and reacting.

FORM (*rūpa*) 1.8, 17; 3.21, 46; the perceptible form by which we recognize something; similarity (*ekarūpatva*) 4.9; sameness (*sārūpya*) 1.4; cf. identity (*svarūpa*).

FOUNDATION, STAGE (*bhūmi*) 1.14, 30; 2.27; 3.6; a basis or grounding; also, a stage or level of yogic achievement; cf. the Buddhist notion of *bhūmi*.

FREEDOM, ABSOLUTE FREEDOM (*kaivalya*) 2.25; 3.50, 55; 4.26, 34; the isolation and liberation of the human spirit from material nature. This liberation is not the extinction of individual existence or a "death wish" in Freudian terms, but a realization of the potency of calm. A comparable idea of liberation is the Jaina notion of *kevalajñāna,* knowledge of liberation; the term *kevalin,* a liberated being, is used of the Jaina saviors, each of whom is known as a Conqueror (*jina*) and Ford-Maker (*tirthaṅkara*).

FRUIT (*phala*) 2.14, 34, 36; 4.11; the result of action; cf. consequences (*vipāka*).

IDENTITY, INTRINSIC FORM (*svarūpa*) 1.3, 43; 2.23, 54; 3.3, 44, 47; 4.12, 34; a significant concept in Indian thought, which has its parallels in Western psychology, referring to one's intrinsic nature and one's role in the world. In Indian terms this world is the cosmos, while in Western psychology the world is society. An "identity crisis" is a chaotic sense of self, a disorientation; in yoga this would involve the identification of one's essential self with the turnings of thought and with material nature. In the psychoanalytic notion of "ego identity," emphasis is on the relation between individual identity and group identity in the individual's development. In the *Yoga Sūtra,* the idea is to realize an identity that is beyond thought, beyond involvement with the world. Cf. form (*rūpa*).

IGNORANCE (*avidyā*) 2.3, 4, 5, 24; cf. *ajñāna.* In Sāṃkhya ignorance is an erroneous form of knowledge, a misconception, especially the misconception that confuses the self with the world. This false knowledge can only be overcome through practice of yoga; cf. the Buddhist concept of *avidyā.*

INDETERMINACY (*anavaccheda*) 1.26; 3.53; indeterminate (*anavacchinna*) 2.31; not being limited or qualified by association with a particular time, place, or other circumstance.

INTELLIGENCE, UNDERSTANDING (*buddhi*) 4.21, 22; the capacity to apprehend facts and ideas, and to reason about them; one of the cognitive faculties that evolve from matter.

INTUITION (*prātibha*) 3.33, 36; knowledge produced without effort, as if it "shines forth" on its own.

INTUITIVE COGNITION (*nirvicāra*) 1.44, 47; knowledge that does not depend on the consideration of objects of experience, in contrast with cognition, which is reflexive (*vicāra*), i.e., involves reflection on such objects.

JOY (*sukha*) 1.33; 2.5, 7, 42, 46; pleasure, happiness, in contrast to suffering (*duḥkha*).

KNOWLEDGE (*jñāna*) 1.8, 9, 38, 42; 2.28; 3.16, 17, 18, 19, 22, 25, 26, 27, 28, 35, 52, 54; 4.31; ignorance (*ajñāna*) 2.34. *Jñāna* is essentially nonconceptual, spiritual knowledge of transcendental reality, as in the *Bhagavad Gītā,* where it is the theme of the fourth section. Cf. *samprajñāta* (1.17), consciously known.

LIMB OF YOGA (*aṅga*) 2.28, 29; 3.7, 8; the eight means of yogic practice. Cf. 1.31 and 2.40, where *aṅga* refers to the limbs of the body.

LORD OF YOGA (*īśvara*) 1.24; dedication to the Lord of Yoga (*īśvara-praṇidhāna*) 1.23; 2.1, 32, 45. *Yogeśvara,* the Lord of Yoga, is a common epithet of Shiva, but in the *Bhagavad Gītā* and related texts, Krishna is also called *yogeśvara.* The identification and role of *īśvara* in yoga varies according to schools of practice and interpretation. At 1.24, *īśvara* is defined as a distinct form of the spirit (*puruṣa*), unafflicted by the forces of corruption, by action, by the fruition of action, or by subliminal intention.

LUCIDITY (*sattva*) 2.41; nature's lucidity or "intelligence"; the pure, lucid quality of nature's perfection; contrasted with spirit (*puruṣa*) 3.35, 49, 55.

MATTER, MATERIAL NATURE (*prakṛti*) 1.19; (in the plural) the primary constituents of nature 4.2, 3; the constituents from which all else is evolved, including *manas, buddhi, ahaṃkāra,* and the five elements. Cf. property (*dharma*).

MEDITATION (*dhyāna*) 1.38; 2.11, 29; 3.2; 4.6; the unwavering attention to a single thread of thought—a continuous flow of the same thought uninterrupted by any extraneous idea. The Sanskrit word *dhyāna,* referring to meditative practices in Buddhism, was translated into Chinese as *ch'an,* which became *zen* in Japanese.

MEMORY, MINDFULNESS (*smṛti*) 1.6, 11, 20, 43; 4.9, 21; defined by Patañjali as "the recollection of objects one has experienced" (1.11). This is comparable to modern definitions of memory as the ability to revive past sensory impressions, experiences, and learned ideas. *Smṛti* in Buddhist texts means "mindfulness" or "awareness." In Patañjali's usage the word seems to combine the ordinary sense of "memory" and the Buddhist notion of "mindfulness."

MEMORY TRACE (*vāsanā*) 4.8, 24; literally "perfume," used to refer to a residue of experience that clings to the individual. The store of these memory traces accounts for behavior that we call "instinctive." Cf. subliminal impression (*saṃskāra*) and subliminal intention (*āśaya*).

MIND (*manas*) 1.35; 2.53; 3.48; one of the cognitive faculties that evolves from matter and is thus material in nature—the others are thought (*citta*), intelligence (*buddhi*), and the senses. *Manas* is the organ of cognition; *buddhi* is the capacity to apprehend facts and ideas and to reason about them; *citta* is the total process of thought.

MORAL PRINCIPLE (*yama*) 2.29, 30; the five universal moral principles that must be undertaken as the first stage of yogic practice: nonviolence, truthfulness, avoidance of stealing, celibacy, and poverty. Together they constitute the great vow that initiates the practice of yoga. Cf. observance (*niyama*), perfect discipline (*saṃyama*).

NONVIOLENCE (*ahiṃsā*) 2.30, 35; taking care not to cause harm to others (one of the five moral principles).

OBSERVANCE (*niyama*) 2.29, 32; one of the eight limbs of yoga, involving personal observances: bodily purification, contentment, ascetic practice, the study of sacred lore, and dedication to the Lord of Yoga.

OBSERVER, THE SUBJECT OF OBSERVING (*draṣṭṛ*) 1.3; 2.17, 20; 4.23; often translated "seer," the one who sees, the seeing subject. The observer is *puruṣa,* the spiritual aspect of everything that is; eye (*dṛś*) 2.6; seer (*dṛśi*) 2.20, 25; the visible world as the object of perception, the phenomenal world (*dṛśya*) 2.17, 18, 21; 4.21, 23; being an object of perception in the phenomenal world (*dṛśyatva*) 4.19; seen (*dṛṣṭa*) 1.15; 2.12. Cf. vision, view (*darśana*).

PASSION (*rāga*) 1.37; 2.3, 7; an emotional response to an experience (especially a pleasant experience) of some external object, which in turn creates a desire for further experiences, thereby binding the spirit to the material world.

PERFECT DISCIPLINE (*saṃyama*), the integrated discipline of *dhāraṇā, dhyāna,* and *samādhi* 3.4, 16, 17, 21, 22, 26, 35, 41, 42, 44, 47, 52; *saṃyama* is the discipline of gaining complete control over the object of contemplation. When *saṃyama* is achieved, the observing self takes the form of the object contemplated, attains complete control over it, and is absorbed in it, obliterating its own nature. Extraordinary knowledge and powers result. In later yogic literature this is called "royal yoga" (*raja-yoga*). Cf. moral principle (*yama*), observance (*niyama*).

PERFECTION (*siddhi*) 2.43, 45; 3.37; 4.1; spiritual perfection entailing the acquisition of supernatural powers.

PERFORMANCE, PRACTICE, ACTIVITY (*kriyā*) 2.1, 18, 36; according to most commentators, *kriyā-yoga,* yoga performance (2.1), refers only to the first five stages or limbs of practice. Patañjali may also be implying a comparison with *karma-yoga,* the discipline of action in the *Bhagavad Gītā,* where all action is performed as sacrifice.

POSTURE, THE POSTURE OF YOGA (*āsana*) 2.29, 46; an effortless, restful positioning of the body, one of the eight limbs of yoga. The lotus posture is the paradigm of all yogic postures: sitting with the spine erect and legs folded to form a steady base.

POVERTY (*aparigraha*) 2.30, 39; renunciation of worldly wealth, one of the five moral principles.

POWER, ACTIVE POWER (*śakti*) 2.6, 23; 3.21; 4.34; power in the sense of capacity, skill, or energy, in contrast with *siddhi,* which for Patañjali is the power that comes from spiritual perfection.

PRACTICE (*abhyāsa*) 1.12, 13, 18, 32; defined by Patañjali as "the effort to hold thought still."

PROPERTY, ESSENTIAL PROPERTY OF MATERIAL NATURE (*dharma*) 3.13, 14, 45; 4.12; cf. the subject that underlies the properties of nature (*dharmin*) 3.14; the "essential-cloud" of pure contemplation (*dharma-megha-samādhi*) 4.29, in which pure contemplation pours its knowledge, as a cloud pours rain, without effort.

PSYCHIC FOCUS, "ONE-POINTEDNESS" (*ekāgratā*) 3.11, 12; (*ekāgrya*) 2.41; cf. "single-threadedness," being intent on only one object (*ekatānatā*) 3.2; cf. unity (*ekatva*) 4.14.

PURITY (*śuddhi*) 2.28 (*aśuddhikṣaya*), 2.41; 3.35; pure (*śuddha*) 2.20; purification (*pariśuddhi*) 1.43; purification is the removal and eradication of the forces of corruption (2.3) from thought by means of yoga.

QUALITY OF MATERIAL NATURE (*guṇa*) 1.16; 2.15, 19; 4.13, 32, 34; everything in material nature is composed of three qualities, which are like energy existing in potential form: lucidity (*sattva*), passion (*ragas*), and dark inertia (*tamas*). Of these, Patañjali is only concerned with lucidity, which is contrasted with spirit; cf. lucidity (*sattva*), property (*dharma*).

REFLECTION (*vicāra*) 1.17; reflexive and intuitive thought (*savicāra-nirvicāra*) 1.44; reflection is a higher form of reasoning, which can consider subtle objects; cf. intuitive cognition and conjecture (*vitarka*).

SEED (*bīja*) 1.25; 3.50; of contemplation (*samādhi*), seed-bearing (*sabīja*) 1.46; without seeds (*nirbīja*) 1.51; 3.8; in most thought, such "seeds" develop into further thoughts.

SENSE FACULTY OR ORGAN (*indriya*) 2.18, 41, 43, 54, 55; 3.13, 47; the physical organs of sense perception, which must be isolated from external stimuli by means of yoga.

SENSE OBJECT, MEANING, PURPOSE (*artha*) 1.28, 32, 42, 43; 2.2, 18, 21, 22; 3.3, 17, 35; 4.23, 24, 32, 34; (*arthatā*) 3.11; (*arthatva*) 1.49; 3.35; (*arthavattva*) 3.44, 47; the objects of the external world toward which our thoughts and desires are directed, so that these objects become distractions from mental stillness.

SENSUOUS REALM, SPHERE OF THE SENSES, OBJECT OF SENSE PERCEPTION (*viṣaya*) 1.11, 15, 33, 37, 44, 49; 2.51, 54; 3.54; (*viṣayatva*) 1.45; (*viṣayavant*) 1.35; the material field in which the sense organs come into contact with their respective objects (as, for example, a field of vision).

SEQUENCE, TEMPORAL ORDER (*krama*) 3.15, 52; 4.32, 33; the material or temporal arrangement of things that creates continual transformations. When this sequence is perceived, such transformations cease.

SPECIFICITY, PARTICULARITY, PECULIARITY (*viśeṣa*) 1.22, 24, 49; 2.19; 4.25; nonspecific (*aviśeṣa*) 2.19; 3.35; specificity is anything that marks a difference or distinction.

SPIRIT (*puruṣa*) 1.16, 24; 3.35, 49, 55; 4.18, 34; the spiritual aspect of anything, which is essentially pure consciousness, as distinct from material nature (*prakṛti*); the fundamental objective of yoga is to isolate the spirit from involvement in nature. In translating the *Bhagavad Gītā,* I used "man's spirit" for *puruṣa* because of the dramatic human context, but since *puruṣa* can refer to all sorts of nonhuman beings, I think "spirit" alone is more suitable to this text. Spiritual abstraction that is isolated from nature occurs in the state of *samādhi. Īśvara,* the Lord, is defined as a distinct form of spirit (1.23–28), the appropriate object of the aspiring practitioner's dedication.

STILLNESS (*sthiti*) 1.13, 35; 2.18; a state of steadiness or fixity (especially of the mind).

STUDY OF SACRED LORE (*svādhyāya*) 2.1, 32, 44; the repetition of Vedic hymns aloud to oneself.

SUBLIMINAL IMPRESSION (*saṃskāra*) 1.18, 50; 2.15; 3.9, 10, 18; 4.9, 27; an impression left in subliminal memory after any experience. The aggregate of impressions accounts for instinctive predispositions, which, according to widespread Indian belief, are carried from life to life in the round of transmigration. Although transmigration may be understood literally, for Patañjali the emphasis is on the psychological dimension of impressions that influences all thought and action. Cf. memory (*smṛti*), memory trace (*vāsanā*), subliminal intention (*āśaya*)—terms that are closely related and in fact often seem synonymous.

SUBLIMINAL INTENTION (*āśaya*) 1.24; 2.12; (*anāśaya*) 4.6; the store of experience that lies dormant in memory and impels an individual to action.

SUBTLE (*sūkṣma*) 1.44, 45; 2.10, 50; 3.25, 44; 4.13; the subtle as opposed to the gross aspect of material things, that which is difficult to perceive and understand.

SUFFERING, PAIN (*duḥkha*) 1.31, 33; 2.5, 8, 15, 16, 34; suffering is the natural result of the unrestrained turnings of thought. As in Buddhist doctrine, ordinary existence is inherently painful. The experience of suffering can be avoided only through the practice of yoga.

SUPPORT, FOUNDATION (*ālambana*) 1.10, 38; 4.11; an object viewed as the cause or condition for knowledge.

THING, SUBSTANCE (*vastu*) 1.9; 4.14, 15, 16, 17; an external object of perception or thought.

THOUGHT (*citta*) 1.30, 33, 37; 2.54; 3.1, 9, 11, 12, 19, 34; (*cittasaṃvit*) 3.38; 4. 4, 5, 15, 16, 17, 21, 23; turnings of thought (*citta-vṛtti*) 1.2; 4.18; *citta* is a combination of *manas, buddhi,* and *ahaṃkāra,* the mental evolutes of matter, and is an extremely sensitive, plastic substance in nature, subject to various modifications.

TRANQUILITY (*prasāda, prasādana*); tranquility of thought (*citta-prasādana*) 1.33; inner tranquility (*adhyātma-prasāda*) 1.47.

TRANSFORMATION, CHANGE (*pariṇāma*) 2.15; 3.9, 11, 12, 13, 15, 16; 4.2, 14, 32, 33; unchangeability (*apariṇāmitva*) 4.18; Patañjali's usage is based on the technical meaning of this term in the Sāṃkhya theory of causation, according to which a given cause is continually transforming itself into effects. This idea is fundamental to the view that cosmic evolution is a complex process in which material nature is always changing (*prakṛti-pariṇāma*), always manifesting its latent possibilities. Transformation or change is a constant manifestation of what is latent in the cause.

TRUTH, REALITY (*tattva*) 1.32; 4.14; that which is essential and real, i.e., not subject to any change.

TRUTHFULNESS (*satya*) 2.30, 36; one of the five moral principles.

TURNING, MODIFICATION (*vṛtti*) 1.2, 4, 5, 10, 41; 2.11, 15, 50; 3.43; 4.18; *citta-vṛtti* is "the turnings of thought," referring to the totality of psychomental modifications, conscious, subconscious, and hyperconscious; cf. activity (*pravṛtti*) 1.35; 3.25; 4.5; inactivity (*nivṛtti*) 3.30; 4.25, 30.

VALID JUDGMENT, VALID MEANS OF JUDGMENT (*pramāṇa*) 1.6, 7; not subject to valid judgment (*apramāṇaka*) 4.16; the methods of obtaining accurate knowledge.

VICTORY, MASTERY (*jaya*) 2.41; 3.5, 39, 40, 44, 47, 48; the attainment of absolute control over a mental process or external object.

VISION, VIEW (*darśana*) 1.30; 2.6, 41; (*ātmadarśana*) 3.32; 4.25; through yoga, the mind may perceive the spirit, just as the eye perceives objects.

WISDOM (*prajñā*) 1.20, 48, 49; 2.27; 3.5; in the words of T. S. Eliot, "the truth that surpasses understanding"; cf. knowledge (*jñāna*).

WILL TO LIVE, CLINGING TO LIFE (*abhiniveśa*) 2.3, 9; a corrupting physical instinct detrimental to the process of spiritual liberation; see corruption (*kleśa*).

WITHDRAWAL FROM SENSUOUS WORLD, WITHDRAWAL OF THE SENSES (*pratyāhāra*) 2.29, 54; the deliberate isolation of each of the senses from external stimuli for the purpose of calming the mind (causing thought to cease).

WORD, LANGUAGE (*śabda*) 1.9, 42; 3.17; the audible expression of thoughts, regarded by Patañjali as an opportunity for confusion and the destruction of contemplative poise (1.42).

SANSKRIT KEYWORDS

abhiniveśa	will to live
abhyāsa	practice
ahiṃsā	nonviolence
ālambana	support
anavaccheda	indeterminacy
aṅga	limb of yoga
aparigraha	poverty
artha	sense object
āsana	posture
āśaya	subliminal intention
asmitā	egoism
ātman	essence
avasthā	condition
avidyā	ignorance
bheda	distinction
bhoga	experience
bhūmi	foundation
bhūta	element

bīja	seed
brahmacarya	celibacy
buddhi	intelligence
citi	consciousness
citta	thought
darśana	vision
dhāraṇā	concentration
dharma	property of nature
dhyāna	meditation
draṣṭṛ	observer
duḥkha	suffering
ekāgratā	psychic focus
guṇa	quality of material nature
hetu	cause
indriya	sense faculty
īśvara	lord of yoga
jāti	birth
jaya	victory
jñāna	knowledge
kaivalya	freedom
karma	action
khyāti	discernment
kleśa	corruption
krama	sequence
kriyā	performance
manas	mind
nirodha	cessation
nirvicāra	intuitive cognition
niyama	observance
pariṇāma	transformation

phala	fruit
prajñā	wisdom
prakṛti	matter
pramāṇa	valid judgment
prāṇa	breath
prasāda	tranquility
prātibha	intuition
pratiṣṭhā	basis
pratyāhāra	withdrawal
pratyaya	concept
puruṣa	spirit
rāga	passion
rūpa	form
śabda	word
śakti	power
samādhi	contemplation
samāpatti	contemplative poise
saṃskāra	subliminal impression
saṃvedana	awareness
saṃyama	perfect discipline
sattva	lucidity
satya	truthfulness
siddhi	perfection
smṛti	memory
sthiti	stillness
śuddhi	purity
sukha	joy
sūkṣma	subtle
svādhyāya	study
svarūpa	identity

tapas	ascetic practice
tattva	truth
vairāgya	dispassion
vāsanā	memory trace
vaśīkāra	control
vastu	substance
vicāra	reflection
vikalpa	conceptualization
vipāka	consequences
viparyaya	error
viṣaya	sensuous realm
viśeṣa	specificity
vitarka	conjecture
viveka	discrimination
vṛtti	turning
yama	moral principle
yoga	discipline

NOTES

INTRODUCTION

1. See Pratapaditya Pal, ed., *Light of Asia: Buddha Sakyamuni in Asian Art* (Los Angeles: Los Angeles County Museum of Art, 1984); and Stella Kramrisch, *Manifestations of Shiva* (Philadelphia: Philadelphia Museum of Art, 1981), especially p. 204. See also Kālidāsa's *Kumārasambhava,* translated by Hank Heifetz as *The Origin of the Young God* (Berkeley: University of California Press, 1985)—for example, 1.54 (p. 30).

2. See Karl Potter, *Presuppositions of India's Philosophies* (Englewood Cliffs, N.J.: Prentice-Hall, 1963), pp. 3–5: "The *yogi* is one who seeks to pass 'beyond good and evil.' "

3. The story of Cūḍālā is found in the *Yogavāsiṣṭha.* See K. Narayanaswami Aiyer, trans., *Laghu-Yoga-Vāsiṣṭha,* 2d ed. (Madras: Adyar Library and Research Centre, 1971), pp. 384–438; and Swami Venkatesananda, trans., *The Concise Yoga Vāsistha* (Albany: SUNY Press, 1984), pp. 333–62.

4. What Patañjali calls ignorance or misidentification (*avidyā*) the Vedānta philosopher Śaṅkara calls *adhyāsa,* "superimposition." In both cases a person erroneously attributes the perceived characteristics of the illusory world to the eternal self, thereby revealing a fundamental ignorance of reality.

5. This idea is illustrated in the famous Buddhist parable of the chariot, which was taught to King Milinda by the monk Nāgasena. See the *Questions of King Menander (Milindapañha),* translated by A. L. Basham, in Ainslie Embree, ed., *Sources of Indian Tradition,* 2d ed. (New York: Columbia University Press, 1988), 1:105–6.

6. For a summary of this debate, see Mircea Eliade, *Yoga: Immortality and Freedom,* 2d ed., translated by Willard R. Trask (Princeton: Princeton University Press, 1969), pp. 370–72. Eliade seems to favor a later date.

7. This association was perhaps suggested by one of the aphorisms. In one of his rare similes, Patañjali compares the posture employed in yoga to "resting like Ananta on the waters of infinity" (2.47; see my commentary on this passage in the translation).

8. Jean Filliozat, *The Classical Doctrine of Indian Medicine* (Delhi: Munshiram Manoharlal, 1965), pp. 22–25. Filliozat's discussion of a symmetry between the legends of Patañjali and of the Buddhist philosopher Nāgārjuna is particularly suggestive in terms of the epistemological radicalism shared by the *Yoga Sūtra* and the *Mādhyāmikakārikā.*

9. *Yoga* does not mean here what it means in later religious contexts. Rather, *yoga,* along with other derivatives of the root *yuj,* "to yoke," refers to the harnessing of horses to chariots and draft animals to carts or plows.

10. See Wendy Doniger O'Flaherty, trans., *Hymns of the Rig Veda* (Harmondsworth, Eng., and New York: Penguin Books, 1981), pp. 137–38.

11. In the Pali Canon, the *Sāmaññaphalasutta* of the *Dīgha Nikāya* amply illustrates the recognition of yogic powers in early Buddhist practice. See William Theodore de Bary, ed., *The Buddhist Tradition* (New York: Modern Library, 1969).

12. See Heinrich Dumoulin, *Zen Buddhism: A History,* vol. 1, *India and China,* trans. J. W. Heisig and P. Knitter (New York: Macmillan, 1988), pp. 13–26; E. J. Thomas, *The History of Buddhist Thought* (Lon-

don: Kegan Paul, Trench, Trübner & Co., and New York: A. A. Knopf, 1933); A. B. Keith, *Buddhist Philosophy in India and Ceylon* (Oxford: Oxford University Press, 1923), pp. 143ff.

13. See Eliade, *Yoga,* pp. 162–99.

14. See de Bary, *Buddhist Tradition,* pp. 16–17.

15. The eightfold path—the practical means for overcoming suffering that is elaborated as the Fourth Noble Truth in the Buddha's first sermon—parallels the eight limbs of Patañjali's yoga. The other important Buddhist idea reflected in the *Yoga Sūtra* is that of cultivating the four attitudes of love, compassion, joy, and impartiality (*maitrī, karuṇā, muditā, upekṣā*), which Patañjali mentions at 1.33. The significance of yoga to the Yogācāra school of Mahāyāna Buddhism is best articulated in the *Laṅkāvatāra Sūtra,* in which the term *citta* is used in a way that recalls its use in the *Yoga Sūtra* and in which the way of the yogi is made explicit. See D. T. Suzuki, *Laṅkāvatāra Sūtra* (London: Routledge & Kegan Paul, 1932; repr. 1956), pp. 252–53.

16. See E. W. Hopkins, "Yoga Technique in the Great Epic," *Journal of the American Oriental Society* 22 (1901): 333–79.

17. See *The Bhagavad-Gita: Krishna's Counsel in Time of War* (New York: Bantam Books, 1986). For a bilingual edition, see *The Bhagavadgītā in the Mahābhārata,* translated and edited by J. A. B. van Buitenen (Chicago: University of Chicago Press, 1981).

18. See Surendranath Dasgupta, *A Study of Patanjali* (Calcutta: Calcutta University, 1920; repr. Delhi, 1989), *Yoga Philosophy in Relation to Other Systems of Indian Thought* (Calcutta: Calcutta University, 1930), and *Yoga as Philosophy and Religion* (London: Trübner & Co., 1924). The first two works are digested in *A History of Indian Philosophy,* vol. 1 (Cambridge, 1922; repr. Delhi: Motilal Banarsidass, 1975), chap. 7, which also serves as a good overview of the development of the Yoga and Sāṅkhya systems.

19. On Sāṅkhya, see Potter, *Presuppositions,* especially pp. 106–11 and 150–53. See also Sarvepalli Radhakrishnan and Charles A.

Moore, eds., *A Source Book in Indian Philosophy* (Princeton: Princeton University Press, 1957), chaps. 12 and 13.

20. Potter, *Presuppositions,* pp. 43, 98–100; Radhakrishnan and Moore, *Source Book,* pp. 425, 453.

21. See Gerald J. Larson, *Classical Sāṅkhya,* 2d ed. (Delhi: Motilal Banarsidass, 1979). Larson reviews the main principles of the system on pp. 7–15 and presents a full interpretation on pp. 154–208. A translation of Īśvara Kṛṣṇa's *Sāṅkhya Kārikā* is appended on pp. 255–77; this text is also translated in Radhakrishnan and Moore, *Source Book,* pp. 426–45.

22. *Sāṅkhya Kārikā* 13. 20–22, 54–55, and 57. See Larson, *Classical Sāṅkhya,* pp. 259–60, 262–63, and 272–73.

23. See "Indian Ideas of the Mind," in *The Oxford Companion to the Mind,* ed. Richard L. Gregory and D. L. Zangwill (Oxford: Oxford University Press, 1987), pp. 357–61.

24. Cf. Spinoza in *De Emendatione:* "The better the mind understood its own forces and the order of nature, the more easily would it be able to liberate itself from 'useless' things."

25. See Barbara Stoler Miller, "The Divine Duality of Rādhā and Krishna," in *The Divine Consort,* ed. by John Stratton Hawley and Donna Marie Wulff (Boston: Beacon Press, 1987); and Barbara Stoler Miller, ed., *Theater of Memory: The Plays of Kalidasa* (New York: Columbia University Press, 1983). Indian poets recognized the unique power and aesthetic potential of the emotions of passionate sexual love. The erotic mood that emerges from such love was expressed in the antithetical modes of separation and consummation. To experience this mood in the interplay of its two modes was considered the height of aesthetic joy. In Indian poetry, an act of remembering is the focal technique for relating the antithetical modes of love-in-separation and love-in-consummation.

By remembering the exquisite details of physical beauty and behavior in love, the lover brings the beloved into his presence, and they are reunited in his mind. Even as a literary convention, then, memory has the power to break through the logic of everyday experience, making visible what is invisible, obliterating distances, reversing chronologies, and fusing what is ordinarily separate. We find this vivid form of remembering and memory of a deeper metaphysical kind working throughout Kalidāsa's plays (most explicitly in the fifth, sixth, and seventh acts of the *Śakuntalā*), and in the *Gīta Govinda* of Jayadeva, translated by Barbara Stoler Miller as *Love Song of the Dark Lord* (New York: Columbia University Press, 1977).

26. Translated in Miller, *Theater of Memory.*

27. Although the titles of these sections appear in most Sanskrit editions, they were probably not part of the original text but a commentator's addition. The traditional titles of the first and fourth sections, *samādhi-pāda* and *kaivalya-pāda,* are drawn from keywords in Patañjali's text, but the titles of the second and third sections, *sādhana-pāda* and *vibhūti-pāda,* are not part of Patañjali's vocabulary. It is not unlikely, moreover, that even the division into four sections is the work of a commentator.

28. See Mircea Eliade, *Shamanism* (Princeton: Princeton University Press, 1964), especially pp. 412–20.

29. For the story of Ṛśyaśṛṅga, see *Mahābhārata* 3. 110–113; translated by J. A. B. van Buitenen in *The Mahābhārata,* vol. 2 (Chicago: University of Chicago Press, 1978), pp. 431–41.

30. For an overview of Indian theories of causality, with particular reference to Sāṅkhya theories of causation, see Potter, *Presuppositions,* ch. 6.

31. James Haughton Woods, trans., *The Yoga-System of Patañjali,* Harvard Oriental Series, vol. 17 (Cambridge, Mass.: Harvard University Press, 1914; repr. Delhi: Motilal Banarsidass, 1966).

TRANSLATION

1. *Citta* is a technical concept in Buddhist psychology. In the *Laṅkāvatāra Sūtra,* a Mahāyāna Buddhist text, *citta* constitutes the ba-

sic concept in the idealistic doctrine that there is no objective reality. Rather, everything is constructed of thought alone (*citta-mātra*).

2. My translation was suggested by Jorge Luis Borges's phrase, "To sleep is to be abstracted from the world" (*Ficciones,* p. 114).

3. Cf. 1.50; 3.9, 10, 18; 4.9, 27.

4. Cf. *Majjhima Nikāya* 1, p. 164; *Visuddhi Magga,* book 4. The Pali terms are *saddhā, viriya, sati, samādhi,* and *paññā.*

5. Cf. *Bhagavad Gītā* 7.10.

6. Cf. *Bhagavad Gītā* 8.13; 17.23; *Kaṭha Upaniṣad* 2.16. The nature of the syllable *AUM* (also written *OM*) is examined in early Upanishadic speculation, most specifically in the *Māṇḍūkya Upaniṣad.*

7. See Barbara Stoler Miller, "On Cultivating the Immeasurable Change of Heart: The Buddhist Brahma-vihara Formula," *Journal of Indian Philosophy* 7 (1979): 209–21.

8. This section bears comparison with Buddhist psychology. See *L'Abhidharmakośa de Vasubandhu,* translated by Louis de La Vallée Poussin (Paris, 1923–26); it is one of the nine *recueillements.* See 8.182, n. 4, for a discussion of Buddhist attempts to distinguish between *samāpatti* and *samādhi.* The two terms are closely related—somewhat less differentiated, in fact, than they are in this section of the *Yoga Sūtra.* See also Franklin Edgerton, *Buddhist Hybrid Sanskrit Grammar and Dictionary* (New Haven: Yale University Press, 1953), under *samāpatti,* pp. 571–72.

9. See the entry on the *Sāṅkhyakārikā* in *Sources of Indian Tradition,* 2d ed., 1:312ff.

10. A central doctrine of Buddhism, *pratītyasamutpāda* more literally means "origination by dependence" of one thing on another. The cycle consists of a circular chain composed of twelve links. From each the next one inevitably arises, binding the individual to the wheel of birth and death. Two basic links are ignorance (*avidyā*) and subliminal impressions (*saṃskāra*), both of which are crucial to Patañjali's teaching. See Ainslie T. Embree, ed., *Sources of Indian Tradition,* 2d ed. (New York: Columbia University Press, 1988), 1:101–3.

11. These five principles—nonviolence, truthfulness, avoidance of stealing, celibacy, and the absence of greed—are also the five vows of Jain spiritual practice.

12. These same principles were the basis of Mahatma Gandhi's nonviolent campaign against the forces of British colonialism, in which every freedom fighter was to use the force of truth (*satyāgraha*) to overcome physical and psychological obstacles. Gandhi also stressed the power of celibacy to focus the energy of the individual.

13. Cf. *Bhagavad Gītā* 2.14, 15, 48, where the equanimity of yoga is defined by impartiality to pairs of opposites, such as failure and success.

14. Cf. *Īśā Upaniṣad* 15: "The face of truth is concealed by a golden disc. O Pūṣan, uncover it, that one who has truth as his dharma may behold it."

15. Cf. *Bhagavad Gītā* 2.41, 44; 6.10, 12.

16. See Stephen Hawking, *A Brief History of Time* (New York: Macmillan, 1988), chap. 10.

17. Cf. *Ṛg Veda* 10.136.4, where the sages (*muni*) are said to move through the air.

18. For a more technical discussion, see Bimal Krishna Matilal, *Perception: An Essay on Classical Indian Theories of Knowledge* (Oxford: Oxford University Press, 1986).

19. My interpretation of these controversial aphorisms has been influenced by that of J. W. Hauer in *Der Yoga* (Stuttgart, 1958) and of Georg Feuerstein in his translation, *The Yoga-Sutra of Patanjali* (Folkstone, Eng.: Dawson, 1979; Rochester, Vt.: Inner Traditions, 1989).

20. The debate about the reality of external objects bears comparison with the Western philosophical positions of Berkeley and Kant.

21. This seems to be a reference to the Buddhist theory of the existence of *dharmas* in the three time periods of past, present, and future. Collett Cox, who pointed this out, suggests that a Buddhist rendering of aphorism 4.12 might read: "The past and future exist in their own nature due to the distinction among the time periods of dharmas."

22. *Dharmamegha* is also the designation of the tenth and final stage (*bhūmi*) of the Bodhisattva's career in Mahāyāna Buddhism. Here, as elsewhere, Patañjali is using Buddhist terminology in a self-conscious way, much as Buddha in his time used Brahmanical terminology to dramatize how distinct his worldview was. See Har Dayal, *The Bodhisattva Doctrine* (London: Kegan Paul, Trench, Trübner & Co., 1932), p. 291; cf. D. T. Suzuki, *The Laṅkavatara Sutra* (London: Routledge & Kegan Paul, 1932; repr. 1956), pp. 14–15.

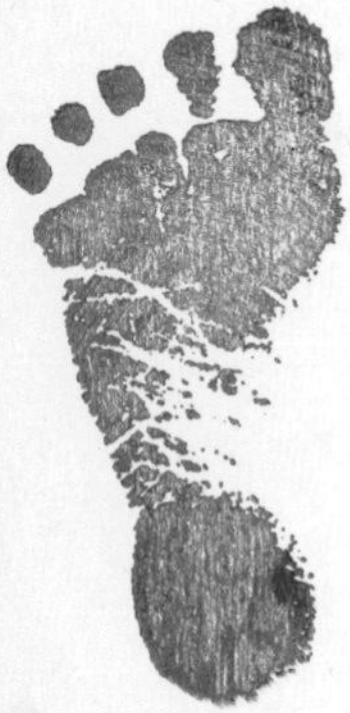

ABOUT THE TRANSLATOR

Until her death in 1993, Barbara Stoler Miller was Samuel R. Milbank Professor of Asian and Middle Eastern Cultures at Barnard College, Columbia University. A leading translator of Sanskrit literature and well-versed in Indian music and art, Dr. Miller edited and translated numerous works of poetry and drama, including her much-praised translation of the *Bhagavad-Gita*. Dr. Miller studied philosophy as an undergraduate at Barnard College and held a doctorate in Sanskrit and Indic Studies from the University of Pennsylvania. She taught at Barnard for twenty-five years.